Successful Practice Learning for Nursing Students

Transforming Nursing Practice series

Transforming Nursing Practice is the first series of books designed to help students meet the requirements of the NMC Standards and Essential Skills Clusters for degree programmes. Each book addresses a core topic, and together they cover the generic knowledge required for all fields of practice. Accessible and challenging, *Transforming Nursing Practice* helps nursing students prepare for the demands of future healthcare delivery.

Core knowledge titles:

Series editor: Dr Shirley Bach, Head of the School of Nursing and Midwifery at the University of Brighton

Personal and professional learning skills titles:

Series editors: Dr Mooi Standing, Principal Lecturer/Enterprise Quality Manager in the Department of Nursing and Applied Clinical Studies, Canterbury Christ Church University and Dr Shirley Bach, Head of the School of Nursing and Midwifery at the University of Brighton

To order, contact our distributor: BEBC Distribution, Albion Close, Parkstone, Poole, BH12 3LL. Telephone: 0845 230 9000, email: learningmatters@bebc.co.uk. You can also find more information on each of these titles and our other learning resources at www.learningmatters.co.uk. Many of these titles are also available in various e-book formats, please visit our website for more information.

Successful Practice Learning for Nursing Students

Kath Sharples

LearningMatters

First published in 2011 by Learning Matters Ltd

British Library Cataloguing in Publication Data
A CIP record for this book is available from the British Library

ISBN: 978 0 85725 315 6

This book is also available in the following ebook formats:

Adobe ebook: 978 0 85725 317 0
ePUB ebook: 978 0 85725 316 3
Kindle: 978 0 85725 318 7

Cover and text design by Toucan Design
Project management by Diana Chambers
Typeset by Kelly Winter
Printed and bound in Great Britain by Short Run Press Ltd, Exeter, Devon

Learning Matters Ltd
20 Cathedral Yard
Exeter EX1 1HB
Tel: 01392 215560
Email: info@learningmatters.co.uk
www.learningmatters.co.uk

FSC
www.fsc.org
MIX
Paper from
responsible sources
FSC® C014540

Contents

About the author

Kath Sharples is Director of Practice and Work-based Learning at the University of West London. Kath's expertise is in developing students' self-regulatory skills in practice learning.

Dedication

To Mum and Dad, with love always.

Acknowledgements

The author and publisher would like to thank the following for permission to reproduce copyright material:

Dennison, B and Kirk, R, *Do, Review, Learn, Apply: A simple guide to experiential learning.* Copyright © 1990, Blackwell Education, Oxford. Adapted Figure 2.7, 'The Johari window', p29, reproduced with kind permission of Blackwell Education, Oxford.

Honey, P and Mumford, A, *The Manual of Learning Opportunities.* Copyright © 1989, Peter Honey Publications, EDI, Coventry, CV3 4PE. Adapted table on 'Conscious learning', p1, reproduced with kind permission of Peter Honey Publications, EDI, Coventry, CV3 4PE.

Honey, P and Mumford, A, *The Manual of Learning Styles.* Copyright © 1992, Peter Honey Publications, EDI, Coventry, CV3 4PE. Adapted learning cycle diagram, p7, and Learning Styles text extract, pp5–6, reproduced with kind permission of Peter Honey Publications. The publisher would like to note that *The Manual of Learning Styles* is now out of print and has been replaced by Honey, P and Mumford, A, 2006, The *Learning Styles Questionnaire: 80-item version*, Peter Honey Publications, EDI, Coventry, CV3 4PE.

Kolb, David A, *Experiential Learning: Experience as the source of learning and development.* Copyright © 1984, p42. Figure 3.1 adapted by permission of Pearson Education Inc., Upper Saddle River, NJ.

Pattison, D, Parsons, D and Weatherhead, C, Connecting reflective practice with clinical supervision, in Ghaye, T and Lilliman, S (eds) *Effective Clinical Supervision: The role of reflection.* Copyright © 2000, Quay Books, Salisbury, Wiltshire. Adapted text extract, p76, reproduced with kind permission of Quay Books, MA Healthcare Ltd.

Every effort has been made to trace all copyright holders within the book, but if any have been inadvertently overlooked the publisher will be pleased to make the necessary arrangements at the first opportunity.

Introduction

About this book

Congratulations on deciding to pursue a career in nursing. The degree you are undertaking will lead to a prestigious professional qualification of which you should be very proud. This book is aimed primarily at first-year pre-registration nursing students who wish to improve their experiences of practice learning. Perhaps you are at the beginning of your degree and wish to prepare for that first experience of being 'in practice'. Or perhaps you already have some practice experience and are keen to improve your practice learning experiences. Whatever the reason, rest assured that this book is for you. Not only is it packed with advice for practice learning, it will also help to allay common fears, and perhaps even correct some misconceptions you may have about the practice environment. This book will be an invaluable tool in ensuring that your practice experiences are the most valuable learning experiences they can be.

Book structure

In Chapter 1, 'What is practice learning?' we begin the learning journey by reviewing a brief history of your pre-registration nursing curriculum. We will explore how and why decisions were made regarding the purpose and nature of practice learning, and the relevant NMC standards that impact upon your practice learning experience.

In Chapter 2, 'How do I learn?' there will be an opportunity to explore the relevance of adult learning theory and learning styles in relation to your practice learning experience. We will delve briefly into the main characteristics of adult learning theory before considering more practical implications for learning, such as your past learning experiences, your learning style, and how your learning style will affect your learning in practice.

In Chapter 3, 'Preparing for practice', we will discuss the specific preparation you will need to undertake prior to the commencement of practice learning experiences. Not only will you have an opportunity to identify the key aspects of practice preparation, you will also be challenged to consider your personal needs and the practicalities involved in planning confidently for your learning experiences.

In Chapter 4, 'Working with my mentor', we will explore the role and responsibility of your mentor in terms of your practice learning experience and assessment of competence. There will be an opportunity to review NMC standards, look at issues related to assessment in practice, and clarify key aspects of the sign-off mentor role.

In Chapter 5, 'Planning my practice experience', we will take a practical approach to the planning of learning experiences. We will investigate how to use an experiential learning cycle in order to plan your practice learning experiences, and how reflection can be used to learn from practice experiences.

In Chapter 6, 'Independent learning in practice', we will develop a clear understanding of the theory behind, and purpose of, self-regulated learning in practice. There will be a chance to explore how independent learning can be developed and the specific challenges of learning in practice. The use of a practice portfolio will be investigated as a means of providing evidence of learning and developing competence.

In Chapter 7, 'Using feedback to learn', the role of feedback in relation to your learning experience and assessment of competence will be addressed. The chapter will be focused on indentifying the key aspects of verbal and written feedback, understanding the relevance of the feedback in facilitating learning, and the role of the mentor in delivering feedback.

In Chapter 8, 'Succeeding in practice', we will identify the role that motivation plays in your practice learning experience, and the potential obstacles to learning that you may encounter. We will discuss various factors that affect a successful practice experience, the difference between intrinsic and extrinsic motivation, and common threats that may stand in your way to success. We will also explore a number of strategies you can use for remaining motivated to learn in practice.

Requirements for the NMC *Standards for Pre-registration Nursing Education* and the Essential Skills Clusters

The Nursing and Midwifery Council (NMC) has established 'Standards for competence' to be met by applicants to different parts of the register, and these are the standards it considers necessary for safe and effective practice. In addition to the competencies, the NMC has set out specific skills that nursing students must be able to perform at various points of an education programme. These are known as Essential Skills Clusters (ESCs). This book is structured so that it will help you to understand and meet the competencies and ESCs required for entry to the NMC register. The relevant competencies and ESCs are presented at the start of each chapter so that you can clearly see which ones the chapter addresses. Each chapter makes links to the *generic standards* that all nursing students, irrespective of their field, must achieve in terms of developing competence in practice learning. This book includes the latest standards for 2010 onwards, taken from *Standards for Pre-registration Nursing Education* (NMC, 2010).

Learning features

Activities

Throughout the book you will find activities in the text that will help you to make sense of, and learn about, the material being presented by the author. Some activities ask you to reflect on aspects of practice, or your experience of it, or the people or situations you encounter. *Reflection* is an essential skill in nursing, and it helps you to understand the world around you and often to identify how things might be improved. Other activities will help you develop key skills, such as your ability to *think critically* about a topic in order to challenge received wisdom, or your ability to *research a topic and find appropriate information and evidence*, and to be able to make decisions using that evidence in situations that are often difficult and time-pressured. Finally, as communication and working as part of a team are core to all nursing practice, some activities will ask you to carry out *group activities* or think about your *communication skills* to help develop these.

All the activities require you to take a break from reading the text, think through the issues presented and carry out some independent study, possibly using the internet. You may find it beneficial to undertake some activities with colleagues so you can learn from each other. Where appropriate, there are outline answers presented at the end of each chapter, and these will help you to understand more fully your own reflections and independent study. Remember, academic study will always require independent work; attending lectures will never be enough to be successful on your programme, and these activities will help to deepen your knowledge and understanding of the issues under scrutiny and give you practice at working on your own.

You might want to think about completing these activities as part of your personal development plan (PDP) or portfolio. After completing the activity, write it up in your PDP or portfolio in a section devoted to that particular skill, then look back over time to see how far you have developed. You can also do more of the activities for a key skill that you have identified a weakness in, which will help build your skill and confidence in this area.

Case studies

Within each chapter there are case studies presented that describe a real-life situation from the practice environment. The case studies have been included so that you may further understand the material being presented. You may wish to discuss and reflect on the case studies with senior students, as they may have experienced similar situations and could provide valuable insights through their experience.

Scenarios

Scenarios are presented in this book to find a fictitious but realistic perspective on the information being discussed. These have been included so that you may develop the skill of thinking about issues from a number of different viewpoints. For this reason, some of the scenarios require you to put yourself in another person's shoes, considering how and why you would react to a given situation.

There are explanations in the Glossary for words in **bold** in the text.

Chapter 1
What is practice learning?

NMC Standards for Pre-registration Nursing Education

This chapter will address the following competencies:

Domain 1: Professional values

1. All nurses must practise with confidence according to *The Code: Standards of conduct, performance and ethics for nurses and midwives* (NMC, 2008a), and within other ethical and legal frameworks. They must be able to recognise and address ethical challenges relating to people's choices and decision-making about their care and act within the law to help them and their families and carers find acceptable solutions.

5. All nurses must fully understand the nurse's various roles, responsibilities and functions, and adapt their practice to meet the changing needs of people, groups, communities and populations.

Domain 3: Nursing practice and decision-making

1. All nurses must use up-to-date knowledge and evidence to assess, plan, deliver and evaluate care, communicate findings, influence change and promote health and best practice. They must make person-centred, evidenced-based judgements and decisions, in partnership with others involved in the care process, to ensure high quality care. They must be able to recognise when the complexity of clinical decisions requires specialist knowledge and expertise, and consult or defer accordingly.

NMC Essential Skills Clusters

This chapter will address the following ESCs:

Cluster: Care, compassion and communication

1. As partners in the care process, people can trust a newly registered graduate nurse to provide collaborative care based on the highest standards, knowledge and competence.

Cluster: Organisational aspects of care

12. People can trust the newly registered graduate nurse to respond to their feedback and a wide range of other sources to learn, develop and improve services.

Chapter aims

The aim of this chapter is to explore the recent developments of the pre-registration nursing curriculum and how this will impact on your practice learning experience.

After reading this chapter you will be able to:

*   identify the key development stages of the current pre-registration nursing standards and competencies;
*   understand the relevance of NMC standards in relation to pre-registration nursing and your practice learning experience;
*   make sense of your pre-registration nursing programme in relation to the structure and content of your practice learning opportunities.

Introduction: starting to learn

Most student nurses begin their nurse training with many questions about their training and very few firm answers. These questions are often regarding the practice learning element of the programme. If this sounds like you, then rest assured you are not alone. Taking any university course can be daunting; however, the nursing course can add a whole new dimension to your stress as the requirement to spend 50 per cent of your training 'in practice' can take you right out of your comfort zone.

Activity 1.1	*Reflection*

Have a look at the list of questions below. Do you know the answers? Have you ever considered these questions before?

*   Who decides what I need to learn to be a nurse?
*   Who decides on the content of my programme?
*   Who makes the decisions about my learning in practice – where I go, what I do and how long I do it for?
*   What will be expected of me in practice?

As this activity is for your own reflection, there is no outline answer at the end of the chapter.

The questions in Activity 1.1 may have occurred to you before, or this may have been the first time you have questioned anything about your nursing course. Don't worry if you do not know the answers to these questions. What does matter is that you find out the answers. This is because your whole nursing programme and, specifically, the practice element of your training is based on the answers to these questions. The aim of this chapter is to begin to answer these initial questions that you may have regarding your practice learning. We will start with a quick history lesson in relation to nurse education, and then we will move on to the role of the NMC in relation to your nursing course. There will be an opportunity to identify the key requirements of your practice learning opportunities and how your nursing programme will have been designed to meet these requirements. There will also be an opportunity for you to investigate your overall nursing programme structure and clarify when practice experiences are likely to occur.

A quick history lesson

In the 1980s, nurse education in the United Kingdom (UK) transferred from hospitals to universities. This decision was made after years of consultation undertaken by the United Kingdom Central Council (UKCC). The grand plan for the future of nurse education in the UK was outlined in a document called *Project 2000: A new preparation for practice* (UKCC, 1986). This was a very dramatic change and caused quite a lot of controversy. Many people were against moving nurse education into universities; however, the decision was made following much criticism of the then methods of preparing future nurses (UKCC, 1999). The reality was that many other countries in the world, such as the USA and Australia, had already moved to university training for nurses. So it was really only a matter of time until the UK did the same. Many people felt that UK nurses would be left behind if they did not adopt the same training approach as the rest of the world. The goal was to prepare nurses for a career of changing roles, lifelong learning and continuing professional development (CPD) (UKCC, 1999). As a result, the apprenticeship style of nurse training was abandoned in favour of university-based education.

Project 2000 involved many important decisions and issues being discussed by the UKCC regarding how nurses were to be trained. One of the issues involved the amount of time that students would spend in theory learning and practice learning. Another issue was related to the role of student nurses during their practice experience. The move into university training meant that student nurses were no longer to be regarded as part of the workforce. However, when the original *Project 2000* curriculum was implemented during the early 1990s, the final 20 per cent of a student's time in practice was known as **rostered service** (UKCC, 1986). As a result, student nurses were counted in workforce numbers.

The implementation of rostered service caused some notable problems. While this approach may have been advantageous in terms of staffing levels, it did not provide student nurses with the best possible learning experiences. Many students found that, instead of being given additional learning opportunities and responsibility, they were more likely to be delegated the role of nursing assistants. As a result, students were finishing their nurse training unprepared for the accountability and responsibility of a registered nurse. In light of this development, one of the key recommendations within the *Fitness for Practice* report (UKCC, 1999) required that students be provided with consistent clinical supervision in a supportive learning environment during all practice learning. This effectively extended the **supernumerary status** for students to include the whole of the programme.

Research summary: Fitness for practice

In 1998, the UKCC undertook an urgent review of the standards for pre-registration nursing and midwifery programmes in the UK. Chaired by Sir Leonard Peach, the Commission for Education was given the following remit:

To prepare a way forward for pre-registration nursing and midwifery education that enables fitness for practice based on healthcare need.
(UKCC, 1999, p6)

The report highlighted that there were numerous problems associated with pre-registration nursing programmes, and that there was disturbing anecdotal and empirical evidence that newly qualified nurses and midwives required constant support, raising questions regarding **fitness for practice** at the point of registration. The report highlighted that problems associated with the organisation and supervision of practice placements, in conjunction with work pressures and the pace of healthcare environments, were hindering the development of practice skills.

As a result, the *Fitness for Practice* report included a number of recommendations for changes to the delivery and structure of practice placements within preregistration nursing programmes. Most notable among a host of recommendations were the following:

Recommendation 10
- *That the standards required for registration as a nurse be constructed in terms of outcomes for theory and practice.*
- *That the standards required for registration as a nurse specify that consistent clinical supervision in a supportive learning environment during all practice placements is necessary.*
(UKCC, 1999, p37)

In addition, the report highlighted that assessment of a student's competence during practice placements could not be reduced solely to an assessment of a student's ability to carry out certain tasks. In other words, there was a requirement for students to demonstrate their competence through work, rather than an emphasis on performance during task-based work. The report saw the birth of a new term; '**knowledgeable doer**' became synonymous with the concept that pre-registration nursing programmes should not only prepare students for fitness for practice at the point of registration, but also should provide them with the higher-order intellectual skills and abilities for life-long learning (UKCC, 1999).

Being supernumerary

The term 'supernumerary' is one of the most controversial and misunderstood terms within nurse education in the UK. Originally, the term was intended to mean that students would be viewed as additional to the numbers of staff already employed in a practice area. Students were given supernumerary status in order to ensure that they were free to learn, and engage with the best and most appropriate learning opportunities for their level of training. It was never intended that students would no longer involve themselves in work while on practice learning. Unfortunately, over time, the meaning of the word has became confused, and students and nurses alike have interpreted 'supernumerary' as implying that students are to observe practice rather than participate in work during practice learning.

The reason for this confusion is unclear; however, this is possibly due to some nurses and students falsely assuming that, as students were no longer to be considered part of the workforce, they would not be participating in 'work'. This misconception still exists in many practice areas today, and some students also continue to perpetuate the myth that they are on practice to observe only. This is quite clearly incorrect, and students who believe this do themselves and their colleagues a disservice. So, once and for all, let's get it clear. According to the NMC:

> *Supernumerary means that the student will not, as part of their programme of preparation, be contracted by any person or body to provide nursing care.*
> (NMC, 2010, p20)

Put quite simply, this means that, as a student, you are to be considered additional to the numbers required to deliver safe nursing care within a practice area. This means that you will have the freedom to learn through work on practice learning. It does not mean that you are to take on an observation role only, as quite clearly it is just not possible to learn in this way.

The significance of the decision to grant students supernumerary status cannot be overestimated. This one decision has had an enormous impact on the learning opportunities and experiences available to you today. The way you learn in practice now, and your opportunities for learning, all stem from the fact that you are supernumerary and, in essence, have been awarded the freedom to learn. The NMC has recently reinforced the supernumerary status of students by clarifying that all your practice experiences should be education-led, with you having supernumerary status for all pre-registration practice experiences (NMC, 2010). We will continue to look at supernumerary status throughout this book, including the ways in which you can use supernumerary status to maximise your learning opportunities. However, for the time being we need to take a closer look at who is currently in control of your nursing programme.

The NMC

On 1 April 2002, the Nursing and Midwifery Council (NMC) replaced the UKCC as the regulatory body for nurses and midwives in the UK (NMC, 2004). As a result, it is now the NMC that decides on the core content of the preregistration nursing curriculum and the overall structure of the programme. Obviously, the main recommendations from the *Fitness for Practice* report (UKCC, 1999) have been revised over the years, although many of the key principles still feature within current programme guidelines. In keeping with this, from time to time the NMC will review their current standards and recommendations for nursing education in the UK. Changes are usually made after consultation exercises that can last many years and are based on feedback from a wide range of sources, including nurses and students. At the moment there is one main document that contains the standards for pre-registration nursing education in the UK.

This document is called the *Standards for Pre-registration Nursing Education* (NMC, 2010), which has now replaced the *Standards of Proficiency for Pre-registration Nursing Education* (NMC, 2004) and the *Essential Skills Clusters for Pre-registration Nursing Programmes* (NMC, 2007). We will need to take a closer look at the new 2010 standards in order to understand all the elements of your practice learning opportunities.

Standards for Pre-registration Nursing Education

The *Standards for Pre-registration Nursing Education* (NMC, 2010) have been provided by the NMC to guide your university on the structure and nature of your nursing programme. They are the current gold standard for how nurses are to be trained in the UK, and set the criteria that all universities must follow. By providing these standards, the NMC is able to control and monitor the quality of the nursing programme you receive. It also ensures that, no matter what university you attend, you will be receiving a pre-registration education programme that is of equal quality for all nursing students in the UK. These standards are not negotiable and your university will have had to provide evidence to the NMC of how your education programme supports the standards they have set.

The *Standards* contain two distinct elements that relate to pre-registration nursing.

- *Standards for education* – the requirements that all pre-registration nursing programmes must meet. These standards include all elements of teaching, learning and assessment of students.
- *Standards for competence* – the knowledge, skills and attitudes that all nursing students need to be able to demonstrate by the point of registration. Most of these competencies are generic across all fields; however, some competencies are specific to the separate fields of pre-registration.

All of the generic 'Standards for competence' set by the NMC are available online. Take some time now to review the generic 'Standards for competence' expected of you in order to register as a nurse.

In addition to these 'Standards for competence', the NMC requires that you will agree to and embrace the code that all registered nurses must uphold before they can enter the professional register. *The Code: Standards of conduct, performance and ethics for nurses and midwives* (NMC, 2008a) requires all nurses to conduct themselves within an ethical framework. As a pre-registration student you will be assessed on these standards in conjunction with the *Guidance on Professional Conduct for Nursing and Midwifery Students* (NMC, 2009). In fact, many of the NMC 'Standards for competence' in the 'Professional values' domain relate directly to professional conduct and ethics within these two documents.

Standards for education

The NMC expects that your university (or approved education institution, AEI) and practice areas will work in partnership to develop, approve and deliver your education programme. For this reason, the NMC refers to 'programme providers' to describe this partnership. From your point of view, it is important to realise that, although you may be based within a university, your practice areas will have made a significant contribution to the design and delivery of your nursing programme.

Standards for education

The NMC has provided a comprehensive list of standards that must be followed in order to provide your nursing programme. These standards are as follows.

1. *Safeguarding the public* – the education of nurses must be consistent with *The Code: Standards of conduct, performance and ethics for nurses and midwives* (NMC, 2008a).
2. *Equality and diversity* – the education of nurses and midwives must be based on principles of equality.
3. *Selection, admission, progression and completion* – these processes must be open and fair.
4. *Support of students and educators* – programme providers must support students to achieve programme outcomes and support educators to undertake relevant personal development.
5. *Structure, design and delivery of programme* – the programme must be developed in partnership using evidenced-based sources to meet approved outcomes.
6. *Practice learning opportunities* – these must be integral to the programme, appropriate to meet the programme outcomes and within a safe and effective environment.
7. *Outcomes* – the programme outcomes must ensure that NMC standards for competence are met and that, on completion, students are fit for practice and fit for award.
8. *Assessment* – programme outcomes must be tested through valid and reliable assessment processes.
9. *Resources* – the educational facilities in academic and practice settings must support delivery of the approved programme.
10. *Quality assurance* – programme providers must have effective quality assurance processes in which findings lead to quality enhancement.

As you can see, the areas covered by the *Standards* are very comprehensive and many of them relate specifically to your experience of learning in practice. The NMC also provides detailed instructions in three forms to explain each of the ten standards:

- *requirements* – which underpin the standards and must be met;
- *guidance* – which should be followed, and reflects what the NMC views as best practice;
- *advice* – which provides additional information but is not mandatory.

The requirements and guidance that provide detail for the standards form part of legislation and, as a result, they must be met.

Activity 1.2   *Reflection*

This activity allows you to check your knowledge regarding the practice elements of your programme. Try to base your answers on your current level of understanding rather than looking it up or asking a colleague. This will help you to gauge what you currently know

continued opposite . . .

continued . . .

and if you have a clear understanding of current practice requirements. As we move through the remainder of this chapter you will be able to reflect on your original answer to check the accuracy of your understanding.

1. A patient/service user cannot refuse to be cared for by a student nurse. Yes/No
2. If you pass all of your practice learning opportunities you will be able to qualify as a nurse. Yes/No
3. I should work with my **mentor** for 40 per cent of each week. Yes/No
4. I will need to complete at least 2,300 hours of practice experience during my pre-registration programme. Yes/No

An outline answer is given at the end of the chapter.

For every aspect of the ten standards your nursing programme is subject to requirements, guidance and advice set by the NMC. As you can imagine, this information is vast and gives explicit detail that must be followed.

In terms of practice learning opportunities, the NMC outlines very specific criteria that must be met. Some of these aspects will obviously play a significant role in your ability to undertake and complete the practice element of your education. Those elements of most significance to you include the following.

- Practice learning experience must provide students with experience of 24-hour and seven-day care.
- Programme providers must ensure that, normally, there are two progression points separating the programme into three equal parts.
- Towards the end of the first and second parts of the programme there is a period of at least four weeks of continuous practice learning.
- Towards the end of the programme there is a period of at least 12 weeks of practice learning.

Case study

Rebecca is a first-year student nurse in the Child field. When she commenced her programme she assumed that she would be able to retain her part-time weekend job in the local supermarket. The university had made it clear that practice experiences would require a 24/7 commitment, but Rebecca assumed that allowances would be made for her personal situation. During her first practice module Rebecca found that there would be a requirement to attend practice on several weekends and she requested that this could be changed. Rebecca was shocked when her request was denied. Her programme leader explained that, in order to meet NMC standards over the three years of her course, she would need to gain experience of practice during weekend periods and also be prepared to attend the same shifts as her mentor. Rebecca decided to resign her permanent weekend job and

continued overleaf . . .

continued . . .

> *seek alternative employment that would allow her to meet her course requirements. She realised that the nursing course had very different requirements from those of any other degree as it was subject to NMC standards in addition to normal university regulations.*

Standards for competence

The NMC does not only produce standards to fulfil educational requirements for your programme. In addition to the 'Standards for education', the NMC also sets the competency standards expected of students as they progress through their pre-registration education. Throughout your nursing course these standards will be used to make judgements regarding your competency. The current standard of competence required of you has been informed by the European Tuning project (Tuning, 2009).

Theory summary: Tuning project

Tuning Educational Structures in Europe started in 2000. Over time, Tuning has developed into a process aimed at (re-)designing, developing, implementing, evaluating and enhancing quality first-, second- and third-cycle degree programmes. Nursing was incorporated into the Tuning project in its second phase, 2002–04. Within the subject-specific document for nursing, a list of 21 competencies at the point of registration was agreed under five different domains. These are:

- *professional values and the role of the nurse;*
- *nursing practice and clinical decision making;*
- *knowledge and cognitive competencies;*
- *communication and interpersonal competences;*
- *leadership, management and team competencies.*

(Tuning, 2009)

Within the *Standards for Pre-registration Nursing Education* (NMC, 2010), the NMC has provided a competency framework that must be used to identify the standard of practice required before a nursing student can apply to be registered. Under this framework you are expected to achieve generic nursing competencies at a minimum of degree level. In addition, you must also achieve field-specific competencies in your chosen field of practice. Once again these must be achieved at degree level.

These 'Standards for competence' (generic and field-specific) are listed by the NMC under the following four domains.

- Professional values.
- Communication and interpersonal skills.

- Nursing practice and decision making.
- Leadership, management and team working.

In addition to simply listing the 'Standards for competence', the NMC also outlines a statement of competence for each domain, which represents a graduate level of competence that has been informed by Tuning (2009). You can expect that these competencies, both generic and field-specific, will be assessed during your practice learning opportunities.

Essential Skills Clusters

In addition to the 'Standards for competence', the NMC has set out specific skills that nursing students must be able to perform at various points of an education programme. These are known as Essential Skills Clusters (ESCs). Within the *Standards for Pre-registration Nursing Education* the NMC (2010) has indicated three different categories of essential skills: those for progression points one and two and those that must be demonstrated for entry to the register. The five essential skills clusters are as follows.

- Care, compassion and communication.
- Organisational aspects of care.
- Infection prevention and control.
- Nutrition and fluid management.
- Medicines management.

Throughout your nursing course you will be assessed according to these standards in both the theory element of your course and the practice element. It is therefore highly recommended that you take the time to read the *Standards for Pre-registration Nursing Education* (NMC, 2010) if you have not already done so.

Activity 1.3   *Evidence-based practice and research*

Take the time now to access and read the *Standards for Pre-registration Nursing Education* (NMC, 2010). While it is a lengthy document, it does very clearly outline the competence expected of you throughout your pre-registration programme. You will be able to put the various elements of your education programme into context and make links between the individual course requirements. By taking the time to absorb this document, you will gain a greater understanding of what may be expected of you during practice experiences and what opportunities there will be for you to learn.

As this answer is based on your own research, there is no outline answer at the end of the chapter.

Learning in clinical practice

It should come as no surprise that the NMC also sets the standards for the support and assessment you receive during your practice learning experiences. The *Standards to Support Learning and Assessment in Practice* (NMC, 2008b) make these expectations very clear, and the majority of your learning experiences in practice will be guided by these standards. We will take a much closer look at these standards and the role of the mentor in Chapter 4. For the time being, though, it is worth noting that these standards exist and that, ultimately, the NMC governs every aspect of your practice learning.

Curriculum design

Curriculum design is a really important aspect of your nursing programme. The course you are doing (or perhaps thinking of doing) was written and designed by a very large team of people – lecturers from your university and also representatives from a variety of practice areas. The process of designing your curriculum will have taken many months and involved many meetings and discussions to ensure that NMC standards were met. The whole of your curriculum will be based on an agreed philosophy of learning and teaching, so that all elements of the programme can be traced back to the same core values. In addition, the curriculum will have been designed to ensure that the requirements outlined by the NMC in the aforementioned *Standards for Pre-registration Nursing Education* (2010) can be met.

Scenario

Imagine that you have just bought a wonderful plot of land and decide to build a brand new house. You start by finding out the building regulations and agreeing the architect's plans. The building work starts with the foundations and then moves on to the general structure. Once these are in place, you add in key features such as walls and floors so that each main section is clearly defined and follows a logical sequence. You gradually add in more and more detail using your own creative style, for example buying furniture for specific rooms and choosing paint colours. When the house is finished it is inspected to ensure that it meets building regulations and complies with the required standards. Once this has been done, it is ready for occupation and you can enjoy it and all its benefits.

Building a nursing curriculum

In some ways, designing a nursing curriculum is a little bit like building a house. The building regulations are like the NMC standards, and the blueprints for the curriculum can be creative, but must comply with the underpinning regulations. The foundations will be based on a philosophy of adult learning, so that all the internal structures of the curriculum are based on that structure. Quite obviously, it is not until you have an understanding of how the whole curriculum will look that you can start to focus on the specific areas. If you tried to build a house by concentrating on the small details first, you would quickly run into trouble, for example furniture that didn't fit the rooms. It is the same principle that underpins a nursing curriculum.

Validation

Once your university and partner practice learning providers had designed the nursing curriculum, they would have asked the NMC for final approval of the course. The NMC would have sent a team of inspectors out to your university to pore over the curriculum plans. They would have looked at all the documentation to ensure that it met their standards and guidelines. When satisfied with the curriculum, the NMC would have validated it. This would have been the final seal of approval that was needed before the curriculum could be taught.

My curriculum

Now that you have an understanding of how your pre-registration course was designed and the elements it must contain, it is important to look at the overall structure of your nursing course. In particular, it is worthwhile for you to understand the structure of your practice learning experiences, where these will be spent and how long you will spend in each one.

Activity 1.4 — *Evidence-based practice and research*

Below, you will find a grid that you can use to document the structure of your pre-registration curriculum. There is an opportunity to outline both the theory and practice elements. Each year is clearly defined so that you can easily identify the individual elements and how these may alter as you progress through the course. Try to include as much detail as possible, for example the module titles, how long each module will be and at what stage in the year it will occur. If you can, include the number of hours you will be required to complete for each module.

Year 1

Module title	Theory element	Practice element

Year 2

Module title	Theory element	Practice element

continued overleaf . . .

continued . . . •••

Year 3

Module title	Theory element	Practice element

As this activity is based on your own observation, there is no outline answer at the end of the chapter.

It is not uncommon to find that some modules will contain no practice element, and some modules will contain no theory. No doubt you will have noticed this when you completed Activity 1.4. However, no matter what the structure or design of your curriculum, you can be assured that it will comply with NMC standards and contain the required elements to expose you to the full range of learning experiences set by the NMC.

The NMC provides, within the *Standards for Pre-registration Nursing Education* (NMC, 2010), very clear requirements that programme providers must comply with when planning your practice learning opportunities. These include a specific requirement that you must have an opportunity to learn in direct contact with healthy or ill individuals and communities (NMC, 2010). The NMC expects that you will be able to use these experiences to organise, deliver and evaluate your nursing care using the knowledge and skills appropriate for each stage of your programme.

The NMC does not dictate the specific types of learning experiences you should have, so there is no requirement for programme providers to stick rigidly to practice areas for a set number of weeks. This means that, rather than a traditional practice placement within a fixed locality, your practice learning opportunity may involve several different locations that may take place across a range of community, hospital and other settings (NMC, 2010). Rather than dictate specific experiences you must have, the NMC allows flexibility in designing your practice learning opportunities that will reflect local and national care delivery approaches, including **care pathways** (NMC, 2010). As we move through this book there will be many opportunities to explore the types of learning opportunities that may be available within these practice experiences.

Chapter summary

In this chapter we looked at the recent history of nursing education in the UK, and the current implications of this for practice learning. The range of standards set by the NMC in relation to the pre-registration curriculum was outlined, along with a brief overview of curriculum design and validation processes. We discussed that, in order to make the most

continued opposite . . .

continued . . .

of the learning opportunities available to you during practice learning experiences, you will need to understand the structure and content of the theoretical and practical aspects of your curriculum.

Activities: Brief outline answers

Activity 1.2 Practice elements of the nursing programme (pages 10–11)

1. The answer is Yes. Under the standard for safeguarding the public, Guidance G1.2.1a states that *Programme providers should consider the impact of student learning on service users and respect their right to decline to be cared for by a student* (NMC, 2010, p8).
2. The answer is No. Under the standard for selection, admission, progression and completion, Requirement R3.11.1 states that *AEIs must ensure that the student has met all theory and practice requirements before they confirm that the programme has been completed successfully* (NMC, 2010, p17).
3. The answer is No. Under the standard for support of students and educators, Requirement R4.2.2 states that *Practice learning providers must ensure that students are supervised directly or indirectly at all times during practice learning by a mentor, practice teacher, or other suitably prepared professional* (NMC, 2010, p19).
4. The answer is Yes. Under the standard for structure, design and delivery of the programme, Requirement R5.2.3 states that *AEIs must ensure that there are at least 2,300 hours of practice learning* (NMC, 2010, p21).

Further reading

Nursing and Midwifery Council (NMC) (2010) *Standards for Pre-registration Nursing Education*. London: NMC.

Available from **www.nmc-uk.org**. Outlines the specific requirements of your nursing course as instructed by the NMC, including the standards of competency you must achieve throughout your training.

Useful websites

www.nmc-uk.org All standards documents listed within this chapter can be easily accessed and downloaded from the NMC website.

Chapter 2
How do I learn?

NMC Standards for Pre-registration Nursing Education

This chapter will address the following competencies:

Domain 1: Professional values

7. All nurses must be responsible and accountable for keeping their own knowledge and skills up-to-date through continuing professional development. They must aim to improve their performance and enhance the safety and quality of care through evaluation, supervision and appraisal.

8. All nurses must practice independently, recognising the limits of their competence and knowledge. They must reflect on these limits and seek advice from, or refer to, other professionals where necessary.

9. All nurses must appreciate the value of evidence in practice, be able to understand and appraise research, apply relevant theory and research findings to their work, and identify areas for further investigation.

Domain 4: Leadership, management and team working

6. All nurses must work independently as well as in teams. They must be able to take the lead in coordinating, delegating and supervising care safely, managing risk and remaining accountable for the care given.

NMC Essential Skills Clusters

This chapter will address the following ESCs:

Cluster: Care, compassion and communication

1. As partners in the care process, people can trust a newly registered graduate nurse to provide collaborative care based on the highest standards, knowledge and competence.

Cluster: Organisational aspects of care

10. People can trust the newly registered graduate nurse to deliver nursing interventions and evaluate their effectiveness against the agreed assessment and care plan.

12. People can trust the newly registered graduate nurse to respond to their feedback and a wide range of other sources to learn, develop and improve services.

Introduction: adult learners

From the minute you enrolled on your nursing course there were certain expectations of you, and assumptions made about you related to your learning. The programme providers that developed your curriculum will expect that you have the ability to be an adult learner and they will have developed the curriculum on the assumption that you will be able to learn as an adult. The implication is that, if you are not prepared to learn as an adult, you may struggle with various learning situations, especially the practice element of your course. It is very important, therefore, to understand the expectations and assumptions of you as an adult learner so that you are able to gain the best possible learning experience during your practice learning opportunities.

This chapter will first consider what an adult learner is, before looking at the main theories and assumptions about how adults learn – assumptions that your course is likely to be based on. We will also look at the factors that may impact on your ability to learn as an adult, investigating how this relates to what will be expected of you in practice. We will then look at how this relates to your own learning style, and what your learning style might be. There will be an opportunity to discover the approaches to learning that suit you best based on your learning style, and how this might be used during your practice learning opportunities. Finally, the chapter looks at what to do if a learning situation does not align with your personal preference.

Can I learn?

In our current culture it is generally accepted that anyone, irrespective of age, has the capacity to learn (Dawson, 2006). While you may agree with this statement, it is worth considering that this belief has not always been held in the past. It was not so long ago that the concept of adult learning was met with some scepticism. There have been numerous myths and misconceptions regarding the impact of ageing and the capacity to learn (Hayes, 2006), and statements such as 'You can't teach an old dog new tricks' have probably perpetuated such myths. However, Withnall et al. (2004) conclude that, while the ability to learn may diminish or be erratic with age, a fit and healthy person continues to learn new things throughout adulthood.

It is important to keep in mind, however, that how you learned as a child does change when you become an adult learner. Adults see the world very differently from the way a child does, and this will affect everything that you do, including the way you learn. The techniques and strategies that you used when you were very young will not automatically work for you as an adult. When you were a child, some of your education would have been focused on teaching you the skills to make learning possible. From an early age you have been exposed to learning how to learn. It is now time to continue this process by learning how to learn as an adult. You will need to develop these skills in order to learn during your practice experiences.

Characteristics of an adult learner

Let us start by looking at some of the characteristics of adult learners.

- *They are above the age of compulsory education.*
- *They have some experience of the world of work.*
- *They have family responsibilities.*
- *They have financial responsibilities.*
- *They have domestic responsibilities.*
- *They are reasonably independent.*
- *They are able to make their own judgements about the world around them.*

(Corder, 2008, pp4–5)

Does this list describe your situation? If so, then you are officially regarded as an adult learner. Being an adult learner does not just focus on your age, but also concerns your relationships, responsibilities and how you relate to the world. The fact that you are an adult learner, however, does not automatically mean that you will have no problems learning as an adult. Just as it was when you were a child, you will need to learn how to learn as an adult. Most importantly, you will need to know how to learn as an adult in practice.

How do adults learn?

So we now know that having the characteristics of an adult learner does not automatically result in the ability to learn as an adult. Over the years there have been many theories about the ways in which adults learn, and the elements within an educational programme that produce the best environment for learning. The specifics of such theories are beyond the scope of this book and will not be dealt with in any great detail. If you want to know more about adult learning theories, there are some suggestions for further reading at the end of this chapter. It is important, however, for you to understand the general principles of adult learning that have guided the development of your nursing curriculum.

The andragogical learner

Your nursing programme will have been designed to meet the needs of the adult or **andragogical** learner. Think back to our housebuilding scenario in Chapter 1 (see page 14). Adult learning theory (andragogy) is just like the blueprint or plans for building the curriculum.

Everything about your curriculum, therefore, is designed to build a nursing course for you as an adult learner. There is nothing new about this approach, as Malcolm Knowles's theory of andragogical adult learning began to gain momentum around the 1970s and continues to be a popular approach in adult learning today.

Andragogy is a term that describes an organised and sustained effort to assist adults to learn in a way that enhances their capacity to function as self-directed learners (Mezirow, 1983). In other words, it is a way of teaching adults that suits the ways in which adults naturally like to learn. At its core, the andragogical approach to adult learning recognises that adults have a unique set of **motivations** for learning (Rogers, 1983). For example, children have very little choice regarding their learning, as education is a legal requirement between certain ages. Adults who are involved in learning, however, are doing so by choice rather than force. No one has made you do your nursing course; you chose to do this for reasons that are important to you. For this reason, the main feature of the andragogical approach is that it encourages adults to use their skills of **self-direction** and their life experiences in order to learn (Howard, 1993). It recognises that adults do not always enjoy being told what to do, and like to use their previous knowledge and experience to work things out for themselves. This means that, as an adult learner, you will be given the opportunity to learn independently in certain areas without the need for constant formalised tuition (Timmins, 2008). As your practice learning experiences will be based on principles of adult learning theory, you should expect that independent learning will feature within your practice learning opportunities.

Scenario

Karl has arranged a trip to a museum. There is an exhibition of Picasso paintings that he has been wanting to see for years. He has been looking forward to this so much that he bought a book on Picasso three weeks ago so that he could understand the background to the paintings selected for the exhibition. He also looked up the museum website and booked tickets to the curator's talk on the paintings. When he arrives he collects an audio guide and takes his time wandering through the exhibition. The book has given him valuable insights into the paintings and the audio guide adds so much more to his experience. The curator's talk is excellent, and he is able to understand so much more of what is said because of his prior knowledge. Karl has enjoyed the whole day and can't wait to share his experiences with his friends.

Can you see that Karl has approached his whole day as an adult learner? He decided to see the exhibition because he was genuinely interested in it. However, he also took responsibility for ensuring that the experience was enjoyable. He did some prior research and arranged to attend a talk. He could have just turned up, as there was no one telling him what to do, but he would have been the one to miss out. By taking the initiative, Karl was able to enjoy and learn far more from the experience.

Assumptions about the adult learner

There has been much debate regarding adult learning theory over the years, but there are five core principles that have remained consistent and are viewed as the gold standard of understanding how adults learn. These in turn have led to some assumptions regarding adult learners. Let us start by looking at these five core principles.

Core principles of adult learning

- *The adult learner wants to be self-directed.*
- *The adult learner accumulates over time a reservoir of experience.*
- *The adult learner has a readiness to learn.*
- *The adult learner is aware of their own learning needs.*
- *The adult learner is motivated to learn.*

(Knowles, 1984, 1989, 1990; Knowles et al., 1998)

It is very important that you understand the significance of these core principles and assumptions about adult learners, as these assumptions will have been made about you. Your nursing course will have been designed based on the assumption that you are an adult learner and that you embrace at least some of the core principles of adult learning. If any of these core principles are lacking, then you may well struggle to learn in the context of an adult learning course.

Activity 2.1   *Reflection*

It is worth taking the time now to reflect on your abilities as an adult learner. Each of the core principles we looked at earlier has been rephrased into a statement about you. Try reading each statement out loud and consider whether this is an accurate description of you.

- I want to be self-directed.
- I have over time accumulated a reservoir of experience.
- I have a readiness to learn.
- I am aware of my own learning needs.
- I am motivated to learn.

If you feel each statement is an accurate statement about you, take the time to write down a brief example of how you have demonstrated this previously in your life. For example, if you feel that you are aware of your own learning needs, write down some brief examples of what these are and how you have identified these needs.

In doing this exercise you will also be building the skill of **reflection**. Perhaps, when you take the time to reflect on specific examples, you may feel that your initial reaction is not accurate. Very often we assume aspects of our character that we may wish to be true but that are not, however, reflective of our current situation. Deep reflection such as this is an invaluable way of understanding more about yourself and your professional development needs.

As this activity is for your own reflection, there is no outline answer at the end of the chapter.

How did you get on in Activity 2.1? Were there any statements that you cannot relate to? In order for each statement to be true, you were required to think of evidence to support each of these statements. For example, how have you demonstrated your readiness to learn? If you are aware of your learning needs, what are they? You see, at the same time as your university may be assuming that you have the qualities required of an adult learner, you may also have assumed that you have these qualities. However, you can't just assume that they exist – there needs to be proof. If you cannot think of examples within each of these criteria, this may be because, at the present time, they do not exist. If this is the case, don't worry – each of these qualities can be learned. This is very good news, as all of these adult learning qualities will be essential for learning in practice.

Positive and negative experiences

While there is no doubt that you are an adult, it may be that you are not yet totally prepared to learn as an adult. There can be numerous reasons for this. It is not uncommon for people to have had negative experiences related to learning. Rogers (2007) suggests that, for some people, their experience of school education has been disappointing and perhaps even associated with ritual humiliation. If this has been your experience, these memories can be quite powerful and can affect your ability to learn as an adult. Dawson (2006) refers to this as the 'baggage' of our previous learning experience.

Not all of your experiences will have been negative, however. There will have been times in your life when you were successful in learning new skills or gaining knowledge. Unfortunately, the memories of negative learning experiences may overshadow your accomplishments. You may feel that you have to repair the damage done from the past before you can learn again (Corder, 2008). In fact, you may be reading this book because you believe that you lack the ability to learn in practice. If your past experiences of learning have been negative, it may be your self-belief that needs an overhaul, rather than your ability to learn.

Case study

Naimh is a mature-age nursing student undertaking a practice learning experience. It has been over 20 years since she last did any formalised study, although she has participated in a number of short courses at an adult learning college in recent years. Naimh begins the experience full of enthusiasm, but she is very nervous as she wants to make a good impression.

In her second week she is attending to the personal care of a client with a learning disability. He is very agitated and begins to hit his head against the bathroom wall. She calls for help and her mentor comes to her aid. The mentor knows the client very well and uses a variety of communication techniques to calm him down. Later on that day, Naimh's mentor asks her if she has been taught any communication techniques during her nursing course. While the remark was not meant to be critical, Naimh feels devastated. She is taken straight back to her school years, when she was accused of being slow and regularly humiliated by teachers. She assumes that her mentor now thinks she is useless and she leaves the room crying, her confidence shattered. Her mentor cannot understand what she has done wrong; she had only wanted to discuss with

continued overleaf . . .

continued . . .

Naimh some communication strategies and had decided to begin by asking Naimh what she had been taught so far on her course.

Naimh has brought into her brand new learning situation painful memories of her past that have not been resolved. The mentor has no knowledge of this, so a simple conversation is interpreted by Naimh as criticism. In order to move on, Naimh will need to make the transition from an adult learning as a child to an adult learning as an adult.

Putting learning into perspective

If your self-belief about your ability to learn has taken a battering over the years, you will need to repair this before you begin your practice learning. If you doubt yourself and lack confidence, you will not be able to make the most of your learning experiences. First of all, please accept and be proud of the fact that, no matter what your educational background or prior experiences, you are capable of enjoying the buzz of learning something new (Corder, 2008). The fact is that we learn all the time, throughout our entire lives. Some learning is formalised, for example at a college or university, and this type of learning may lead to a qualification. Quite a lot of learning that you do, however, may be informal, and you may not even recognise it immediately as learning. It is very easy to trivialise this type of learning, assuming that it doesn't matter, or is not as important or as impressive as the formal types of learning. All learning is important, however, and every time you learn something new you prove to yourself that all learning is possible for you.

Activity 2.2	*Decision-making*

Have a think about the range of skills that you already have, that you learned as an adult. Now use the box below to note down all of these skills. Be honest about your accomplishments and don't belittle yourself. For example, you may be able to rewire a plug or knit a scarf. Perhaps you can repair a bicycle puncture or create a play list on your iPod. It doesn't matter how trivial you may think your achievement is, the fact is you have learned something, so be proud and write it down.

Skills that I have learned:

continued opposite . . .

continued . . .

In deciding upon your list of skills you will need to think very clearly about what makes you unique to others. It is an opportunity to be clear about your skills and the talents you have that others may not possess. There are no right or wrong answers here, but you will need to consider a range of areas within your life in order to decide on the skills that you developed as an adult.

As this activity is based on your own observation, there is no outline answer at the end of the chapter.

Take a very good look at all the things you have written in Activity 2.2. You had to learn all these skills. Over the course of your life you have continued to develop and learn new skills, and every time you add another thing to the list you prove to yourself that you can learn and, more importantly, can learn as an adult.

Adult learning in practice

Without question, there will be certain expectations of you when you undertake practice learning experiences. First, it will be expected that you will possess at least some ability to learn as an adult. You can, therefore, expect to be treated as an adult learner, with the ability to be self-directed and self-motivated in your learning experiences. As a result, your opportunities to engage with the best possible learning experiences will depend on your ability to be self-directed and self-motivated. Do not worry if you are unsure about what this means or how to go about doing it, as there are chapters in this book that will deal with all these issues. At this stage, all you really need to do is understand why these expectations exist.

Second, you can expect to have mutual responsibility for planning your own learning, rather than it being planned for you. Unlike learning that you may have experienced as a child, you will not always be given specific instructions for every learning experience. It will be assumed that you will be able to seek out and plan some of your learning experiences independently. This may come as quite a culture shock, especially if this is your first exposure to an adult educational programme (Knowles et al., 2005).

The focus of this book, therefore, will be on how to develop the skills of an adult learner in practice. Remember that, in order to qualify as a nurse, you will need to demonstrate that you are competent in practice, and practice learning will be the proof of your competence. As we discovered in the last chapter, the *Standards for Pre-registration Nursing Education* (NMC, 2010) make the expectations for your competence very clear. For this reason it is necessary not only to understand that you have the ability to learn, but also to explore how to learn and gain the most during each learning experience. In fact, many of the 'Generic competencies' outlined by the NMC refer directly to a requirement that you are able to acquire new knowledge. In order to do this you will need to uncover and understand your own unique learning style.

Learning styles

The first thing to understand about the way you learn is that it is unique to you. This is generally referred to as your 'learning style' and is linked to various aspects of learning, such as the way you concentrate, process, internalise and remember new information (Dunn and Dunn, 1999). In fact, because the way you learn is a part of your personality, it would be very unusual for your learning style to exactly match someone else's. This also means that the way you learn, the way that works best for you, has developed over many years, although you probably were not aware that it was happening.

Lifelong learning

Throughout your life you have been learning; in fact, not a day goes by when you don't learn something new. Activity 2.2 should have helped you to understand just how many things you have learned as an adult. Sometimes what you learn may take place entirely by chance. Perhaps you listen to the weather forecast and learn about isobars. You may not even be aware that you have learned something, as very often we do not recognise these informal situations as learning. At other times you may deliberately set out to learn something, for example by joining a workshop on Italian cooking. In these situations you will be aware that you are learning, but because it is for pleasure you may feel differently about this type of learning than previous experiences of formal education. However, no matter what situation you learn in, you will bring to that event your individual learning style.

Activity 2.3   *Critical thinking*

The point of this activity is to help you understand that learning happens all the time and is based on the experiences that happen to you throughout the day. You don't have to go out of your way to learn something new. The grid below represents the range of different learning opportunities you may encounter, at university and outside, both consciously and unconsciously, in the course of each day. Now think about the types of learning you have done over the last week, and where and how this has taken place. Use the grid to record some examples of different learning experiences you have had. There is an example in each category to get you started.

Conscious learning at university	**Unconscious learning at university**
• I learned how to take a patient's blood pressure.	• I learned that the lift in B block doesn't stop on the seventh floor.

continued opposite . . .

---

continued . . .

Conscious learning at home and socially	Unconscious learning at home and socially
• I learned how to burn a CD on my laptop.	• I learned that orchids will die if they are overwatered.

Source: Adapted from Honey and Mumford (1989, p1)

As this activity is based on your own observation, there is no outline answer at the end of the chapter.

Take some time to look at the different learning experiences that you have noted in Activity 2.3. It should be obvious that most of the learning that you do comes directly from your experiences. Sometimes your experiences may be purely accidental and unconscious; however, this does not mean that learning through these experiences is any less valid than deliberate, conscious learning (Honey and Mumford, 1989).

Choosing your learning experiences

It is human nature to gravitate towards experiences that you enjoy, and avoid experiences that you do not enjoy. During your practice learning experiences you will be presented with a range of potential learning opportunities, for example practical activities, observation of role models or interacting with people (Harvey and Vaughan, 1990). The point is that you will have a natural tendency towards filtering the range of potential learning opportunities, selecting those that you enjoy and avoiding those that you dislike. As the majority of learning comes through experiences, what and how you learn is largely dependent on the experiences that you choose to engage with. This is particularly true of the unconscious, accidental learning that you do. As a result, your personal likes and dislikes will have a significant impact on the learning experiences available to you.

Case study

Geri lives in London and often drives to Dorset to visit her niece. Geri dislikes driving on major roads as she was involved in a serious motorway accident just after receiving her licence. She prefers to travel on A and B roads for the journey, even though it takes her a little longer. Over the years Geri has worked out her favourite routes, and she now looks forward to travelling through all the different villages and stopping for lunch in a pub along the way. She even allows more time, so that she can make a detour to a farm shop that sells her favourite homemade boysenberry cheesecake. Geri has become a very experienced country driver and has learned a range of alternative routes she can take if there are traffic delays. Geri did not plan to learn these skills; they simply developed as a result of her choices and the experiences she has had.

Understanding your own learning style

The best way to make the most of all potential learning opportunities available to you is to understand your own particular learning style. An appreciation of what makes you 'tick' and the diversity of learning styles among individuals can be the first step towards understanding what types of learning situations will work best for you (McMillan and Dwyer, 1990). It may even explain why you have either consciously or unconsciously chosen or rejected previous experiences. Kolb (1984) suggests that there is a strong relationship between how people learn and how they respond to life situations. It is, therefore, important to recognise your own personality traits and how they contribute to your unique learning style.

Different learning styles

There is a vast range of personality and learning style tests that can help you to understand your own particular style of learning. Before you start this process of discovery, it is important to recognise that no one learning style is any better or worse than any other. There are no right or wrong answers here. There is also a wide range of tests that explore learning styles. The majority of these tests come in questionnaire form and are quite easy to complete. Some tests use personality traits to measure learning preferences. The Myers-Briggs type indicator is one such test (Myers et al., 1998) and discusses four different dichotomies of personality in relation to learning style. Myers (1995) suggests that understanding a student's learning preference can explain why a learner may enjoy and do well at a particular activity. Logic would suggest that the existence of certain personality traits may also explain why a student avoids or does not do well at the opposite types of learning activities.

Other learning style tests are more focused on particular attributes of learning rather than broader determinants of personality, although where one begins and the other ends is almost impossible to unravel. The Learning Styles Questionnaire, developed by Honey and Mumford (1992), is one such tool that can be used for identifying your learning style. The four different learning styles explain not only a preference for a style of learning, but also personality traits that explain preferences for certain experiences over others. It is worth looking at each of the different styles as you may recognise some attributes to be an accurate description of you – both your likes and your dislikes.

Honey and Mumford learning styles

Activists

Activists involve themselves fully and without bias in new experiences. They enjoy the here and now and are happy to be dominated by immediate experiences. They are open-minded, not sceptical, and this tends to make them enthusiastic about anything new. Their philosophy is 'I'll try anything once.' They tend to act first and consider the consequences afterwards. Their days are filled with activity. They tackle problems by brainstorming. As soon as the excitement from one activity has died down, they are busy looking for the next.

thrive on the challenge of new experiences but are bored with implementation and longer term consolidation. They are gregarious people constantly involving themselves with others but, in doing so, they seek to centre all activities around themselves.

Reflectors

Reflectors like to stand back and ponder experiences and observe them from many different perspectives. They collect data, both first hand and from others, and prefer to think about it thoroughly before coming to any conclusion. The thorough collection and analysis of data about experiences and events is what counts so they tend to postpone reaching definitive conclusions for as long as possible. Their philosophy is to be cautious. They are thoughtful people who like to consider all possible angles and implications before making a move. They prefer to take a back seat in meetings and discussions. They enjoy observing other people in action. They listen to others and get the drift of the discussion before making their own points. They tend to adopt a low profile and tend to have a slightly distant, tolerant, unruffled air about them. When they act it is part of a wide picture which includes the past as well as the present and others' observations as well as their own.

Theorists

Theorists adapt and integrate observations into complex but logically sound theories. They think through problems in a vertical, step by step logical way. They assimilate disparate facts into coherent theories. They tend to be perfectionists who won't rest easy until things are tidy and fit into a rational scheme. They like to analyse and synthesise. They are keen on basic assumptions, principles, theories, models and systems thinking. Their philosophy prizes rationality and logic. 'If it's logical it's good.' Questions they frequently ask are: 'Does it make sense?' 'How does this fit with that?' 'What are the basic assumptions?' They tend to be detached, analytical and dedicated to rational objectivity rather than anything subjective or ambiguous. Their approach to problems is constantly logical. This is their 'mental set' and they rigidly reject anything that doesn't fit with it. They prefer to maximise certainty and feel uncomfortable with subjective judgements, lateral thinking and anything flippant.

Pragmatists

Pragmatists are keen on trying out ideas, theories and techniques to see if they work in practice. They positively search out new ideas and take the first opportunity to experiment with applications. They are the sort of people who return from management courses brimming with new ideas that they want to try out in practice. They want to get on with things and act quickly and confidently on ideas that attract them. They tend to be impatient with ruminating and open-ended discussions. They are essentially practical, down to earth people who like making practical decisions and solving problems. They respond to problems and opportunities 'as a challenge'. Their philosophy is: 'There is always a better way' and 'If it works it's good.'

(Honey and Mumford, 1992, pp5–6)

What's my style?

No doubt you will have indentified that you possess certain characteristics of all learning styles; however, there may be one particular style that describes you best. It is quite common to have several attributes of a particular learning style for which you have a strong preference and, conversely, few attributes of a learning style with which you feel less comfortable. As your learning style has quite a lot to do with your personality, you will no doubt see similarities between your learning style and your general likes and dislikes in life.

Activity 2.4   *Critical thinking*

Take the time now to list your learning styles in order – from what you feel is the most like you, to the style that you feel is least like you.

The learning style that is most like me	
The learning style that is somewhat like me	
The learning style that is a little like me	
The learning style that is least like me	

Rather than just list these learning styles, try to think of some recent learning experiences that you have encountered that support your choice. For example, if you feel that your strongest learning style is as an activist, you will need to analyse your role and actions in a variety of learning situations in order to substantiate this. If after your analysis of the learning event your actions support the attributes of an activist, you have possibly identified your most dominant learning style. If you have reacted differently within learning situations, it is likely that you have more than one dominant learning style.

As this activity is based on your own observation, there is no outline answer at the end of the chapter.

Learning and your learning style

While understanding your learning style is an interesting process in itself, it is also invaluable in developing your ability to learn and engage with a wide variety of learning experiences. As we have already discovered, some types of learning experiences are geared towards particular styles of learning, so it is likely that you will gravitate towards learning activities that match with your learning style (Honey and Mumford, 1995).

This is especially important when it comes to learning during practice experiences. There will be a wide range of learning opportunities available to you; however, depending on your learning style, you may avoid the types of experiences that do not match your learning style. You may not always be aware that you are doing this, especially if you are in a situation where learning is accidental. In fact, if you always select learning experiences that you naturally enjoy, you will be very unlikely to engage 'accidentally' with learning experiences that you don't enjoy. In other words, if there is a mismatch between the learning experience and your learning style, you are much less likely to learn, as you will be limiting your overall learning opportunities.

Case study

Trevor is in his third year of his pre-registration programme and making plans for undertaking his final practice experience. He is looking forward to qualifying as a Registered Mental Health Nurse and hopes to specialise in eating disorders. He chooses a specialist eating disorders service as his final practice experience. During the first week Trevor is allocated a small caseload and begins to work with a range of clients. As a theorist, Trevor has always preferred to read through clients' notes and local policies on emergency situations rather than participate in person. On his second day of practice Trevor enters the day room and finds one of his clients self-harming with a razor. Trevor panics and his mind goes blank – he has never encountered a situation like this before. He forgets all about the emergency procedures and instead freezes for a few moments before bolting from the room. In a state of panic Trevor runs from room to room looking for someone to help. Eventually Trevor raises the alarm and staff run to the day room.

Without realising it, Trevor has distanced himself from learning how to cope with situations where an urgent response is required to ensure client safety. Trevor has always relied on and referred to his mentor during previous emergency situations. In doing so he has missed the opportunity to learn how to cope with an emergency and this has led to a serious incident. Trevor realises far too late that his reluctance to involve himself in all learning experiences has not only compromised his competence, but also resulted in his client coming to serious harm.

Does age matter?

We already know that age is no barrier to learning. In fact, older learners form the most rapidly growing segment of the learning population in most Western nations (Delahaye and Ehrich, 2008). While it is generally accepted that older learners may not be as quick to learn as younger learners, Crawford (2004) points out that they more than make up for this through a wealth of experience that supports better reasoning and judgement skills. Thus, while your preferred learning style and the way you learn might change as the years progress, age alone is no barrier to learning.

Learning styles and activities

Table 2.1 overleaf represents some of the learning activities that you may come across during your practice learning experiences. The types of activities are grouped together according to the different learning style profiles they may appeal to.

Matching your learning style with opportunities

You can see from Table 2.1 that there will naturally be some activities that may match certain learning styles better than others. However, you should also be able to see that avoiding certain learning activities because they do not match a particular style could be a potential problem. Remember that the NMC has determined the competence level required of you throughout your training and at the point of registration (NMC, 2004, 2007). If you avoid learning situations simply because they do not match your learning style, you may also encounter difficulties in achieving competence.

Learning style	Learning activities
Activist	• Care of critically ill patients • Bed management issues • Wound care • Diffusing conflict • Emergency situations • Home visits
Reflector	• Developing and following protocols • Multidisciplinary team (MDT) meetings • Ward rounds • Record keeping • Handover
Theorist	• Discharge planning • Drug calculations • Use of risk assessment tools • Care planning • Reviewing/updating policies
Pragmatist	• Airway management • Pre- and post-operative care • Infection control procedures • Medication administration • Referrals to community services • Case conferences • Group therapy

Table 2.1: Learning styles and activities

Case study

Abosede and Siobhan are second-year students. They have been on a community practice learning experience at a health centre for two weeks. Every morning the community nurses meet to discuss the clients they will be treating throughout the day, and to make decisions about new referrals. Abosede has come to dread these meetings. The discussions seem to go on too long and she finds it difficult to pay attention to what everyone is saying. She feels that the meeting is a waste of time as, being an activist, she just wants to involve herself with delivering patient care. She finds she learns most when she is able to discuss each client's needs with her mentor between each visit. Siobhan enjoys the morning review and always listens attentively. She is a reflector and finds it useful to make notes about each client so she can ask her mentor about the various points that were discussed.

continued opposite . . .

continued . . . .

> *In the third week, Abosede and Siobhan are asked if they would like to take on a small client caseload and they both respond enthusiastically. The following day, at the morning review, Abosede is asked to update the team on her clients. She feels under enormous pressure as everyone is looking at her expectantly. She realises that she doesn't know what to say. Her mentor has to look through her case notes to update the team. Siobhan is also asked to update the group and uses her notes to structure a very detailed report. All eyes are on her and she feels proud to be able to discuss her clients with the team and participate in care planning. Abosede leaves the meeting feeling very upset; she knows her clients well, but didn't know how to report during the meeting.*

You will need to make a concerted effort to engage with all learning opportunities, not only those that you naturally enjoy. The good news is that you can develop skills in your least preferred learning style, although it will take some effort and work on your part. Ideally, you should discuss your learning style with your mentor, looking at the types of activities that you most enjoy and establishing a combination of styles that can be incorporated into your learning (Haidar, 2007). Have a look again at Activity 2.4 on page 30 and the learning style that you have the least preference for. There will be very good reasons why this style of learning does not appeal to you; however, in order to make the most of all learning opportunities that come your way, you will need to develop your skills in utilising the full range of learning styles. A starting point is to understand why all learning styles will be important during your practice experience.

Why do I need to be an activist?

If your least preferred learning style is 'activist', it is likely that you will not enjoy learning when it involves a new experience or where there are fresh problems to solve. This will create some difficulties for you in your nurse training as there will be times when action is required and you will need to 'think on your feet'. For example, emergency situations or rapid changes in a patient's clinical condition will require you to make fast and competent decisions as part of a team. This is not the time be slowly thinking through problems or deliberating over the best course of action. Crucially, a part of your learning will be to demonstrate that you can act and react under pressure. Trevor had this very problem in the case study we looked at earlier.

Why do I need to be a reflector?

If your least preferred learning style is 'reflector', it is likely that you will not enjoy learning experiences that involve observing problems or thinking through previous experiences. You will probably not enjoy investigating different types of research and ideas, and may even feel that these activities are a waste of time. However, to demonstrate competence as a nurse you will need to be aware of best practice guidelines and take time to explore alternatives that support evidence-based practice. For example, new wound care techniques or drug therapies may require changes to your clinical practice.

Why do I need to be a theorist?

If your least preferred learning style is 'theorist', it is likely that you will not enjoy spending time over decisions, or lengthy discussions about the best course of action. You may find attention to detail tedious and become frustrated if you cannot get the answer straight away. However, such skills are vital for nurses when you are required to make a complex drug calculation or read carefully through case notes and previous treatment plans. There will be occasions when you will need to take the time to think through problems carefully before acting.

Why do I need to be a pragmatist?

If your least preferred learning style is 'pragmatist', it is likely that you will not enjoy trying out new techniques, or changing the way you do things. You may not be particularly interested in the consequences of actions or outcomes of events. However, 'pragmatic' skills are essential, as these activities are strongly linked to evidence-based practice and to being able to adapt and change patient care plans so that the best treatment options are delivered. This could include a range of activities, from monitoring fluid and electrolyte balance to re-evaluating a discharge plan.

Learning styles and competence

The simple fact is that you will need to use a range of learning styles in order to develop the competence required of a registered nurse. It just will not be possible to avoid using the full range of learning styles, as you will miss out on learning experiences that are vital for your professional development. Li et al. (2008) comment that the development of new skills and knowledge requires a variety of teaching methods and also learning strategies. Don't worry too much at this stage if you come across a particular learning style that you may struggle with, as we will be looking at practical solutions later in the book.

Chapter summary

While everyone has the ability to be an adult learner, it is also true that not all adults will be prepared to learn as adults. It may be that there is a need to overcome negative learning experiences from the past in order to develop the skills of an adult learner. Throughout your nursing course it will be expected that you are able to learn as an adult. You must come to terms with the assumptions and expectations of you as an adult learner in order to develop your ability to learn in, through and during practice. This may require you to develop your motivation and self-direction in practice. In addition, you must understand your own learning style in order to gain the most from each learning experience. Of equal importance, however, is the need to understand the style of learning in which you are weak or may choose to avoid. The learning opportunities that will be available to you in practice will require that you develop a range of learning styles and techniques, not just those with which you are comfortable and familiar. Competence as a nurse will require a mix of learning styles, in equal and proportional measure.

Further reading

Crawford, D (2004) The role of aging in adult learning: implications for instructors in higher education. *New Horizons for Learning*. Available online at **www.newhorizons.org/lifelong/higher_ed/crawford. htm**.

This is a useful essay that looks at the links between ageing, experience, self-esteem and the ability to learn. The particular needs of adult learners are discussed in terms of course content and design.

Dawson, C (2006) *The Mature Student's Study Guide*. Oxford: How To Books.

This book offers some great advice and tips for studying as an adult.

Knowles, M, Holton, E and Swanson, R (1998) *The Adult Learner* (5th edn). Houston, TX: Gulf.

This is a useful text for explaining in detail the principles and application of adult learning theory.

Useful websites

www.mind.org.uk/help/diagnoses_and_conditions/increase_your_self_esteem

This booklet explains the fundamentals of poor self-esteem and reasons that self-esteem may fluctuate and, most importantly, offers some practical advice for improving your self-esteem.

www.peterhoney.com

This website allows you to access a variety of Honey and Mumford learning style questionnaires online; however, you will need to pay for them. There is also the option to buy questionnaires in printed form for individuals and groups.

The internet is awash with different types of learning style questionnaires and the following provide just a small sample of the different options available.

www.learning-styles-online.com/inventory/questions.asp

www.engr.ncsu.edu/learningstyles/ilsweb.html

www.vark-learn.com/english/page.asp?p=questionnaire

Chapter 3
Preparing for practice

NMC Standards for Pre-registration Nursing Education

Domain 1: Professional values

8. All nurses must practice independently, recognising the limits of their competence and knowledge. They must reflect on these limits and seek advice from, or refer to, other professionals where necessary.

Domain 2: Communication and interpersonal skills

3. All nurses must use the full range of communication methods including verbal, non-verbal and written, to acquire, interpret and record their knowledge and understanding of people's needs. They must be aware of their own values and beliefs and the impact this may have on their communication with others. They must take account of the many different ways in which people communicate and how these may be influenced by ill health, disability and other factors, and be able to recognise and respond effectively when a person finds it hard to communicate.

5. All nurses must use therapeutic principles to engage, maintain and, where appropriate, disengage from professional caring relationships, and must always respect professional boundaries.

NMC Essential Skills Clusters

This chapter will address the following ESCs:

Cluster: Organisational aspects of care

10. People can trust the newly registered graduate nurse to deliver nursing interventions and evaluate their effectiveness against the agreed assessment and care plan.

16. People can trust the newly registered graduate nurse to safely lead, co-ordinate and manage care.

> **Chapter aims**
>
> The aim of this chapter is to assist you with understanding the specific preparation you will need to undertake prior to the commencement of your practice experiences.
>
> After reading this chapter you will be able to:
>
> * identify the key aspects of practice preparation;
> * consider the relevance of specific practice preparation in terms of your personal needs;
> * plan confidently for your learning experiences.

Introduction: putting practice learning opportunities in perspective

Given that you will spend at least 2,300 hours learning in practice, it is important that you make the most of this time. Preparation for your practice learning experiences is essential for success. Get your preparation right and each learning experience could be one of the most rewarding and motivating parts of your training. You will have the opportunity to put your brand new skills into practice and link classroom theories with real patient experiences. However, get your preparation wrong and your practice experiences could quickly become times of misery and anxiety. Not only could you become easily discouraged, but you may also jeopardise your performance for practice assessment. The great news is that you can take much of the stress and anxiety out of practice learning simply by preparing yourself for the experience.

Throughout this chapter you will have the opportunity to investigate the essentials of practice preparation. We will start by looking at the major concerns related to practice learning and how to prepare yourself and plan for a learning experience rather than a working experience. The role of your mentor will also be considered. We will then look at the importance of practical aspects of preparation, such as travel arrangements and juggling other work commitments. The chapter will conclude with a checklist for your practice learning experiences and an opportunity to consider solutions to problems you may encounter.

Feelings prior to practice learning

If you are feeling particularly anxious or concerned about your practice experience, rest assured that this is normal, as even students who appear calm and confident may be feeling very nervous on the inside. You have every right to feel this way because many things will be out of your control while in the practice setting. Sometimes this lack of control and fear of the unknown can lead to high levels of anxiety, especially before the practice experience begins (Beck, 1993). One of the key aspects of preparing for practice learning is to acknowledge what worries you the most. You may be concerned about whether you will like the practice area, or if the staff will like you.

Having these fears and concerns is totally reasonable, as the practice environment can be an incredible mix of unpredictable, uncontrollable, challenging and stressful situations (Yong, 1996). A starting point, therefore, is to find out what it is that concerns you. Once you have acknowledged what your fears are, you can start to plan for how you will deal with these situations if they arise.

Activity 3.1	*Reflection*

This list includes some of the typical feelings that past students have felt before their practice experiences. You might find it useful to put a tick next to the ones that apply to you. There are some blank boxes in which you might like to write any other feelings you have.

I'm worried that . . .

I won't fit in.	
the people I meet might think I'm stupid.	
it will feel like I'm being thrown in at the deep end.	
I might seem too slow.	
I won't like my mentor, or they won't like me.	
too much might be expected of me.	
I won't get a chance to practise my skills.	
I won't remember everything.	
I might get left alone with a patient and won't know what to do.	
I might hurt someone.	

Take some time now to look at what your main concerns are.

- Is there anything that you are particularly worried about?
- Are your concerns based on a previous experience, or not related to anything in particular?

You may like to make a quick note as to why you are feeling this way, as we will refer back to this list at the end of the chapter.

As this activity is for your own reflection, there is no outline answer at the end of the chapter.

Preparing for success

If you are preparing for practice learning for the very first time, there is no doubt that this is a momentous event. Students just like you have described their feelings in the time leading up to their first practice experience as a mix of excitement, fear and ambivalence (Gray and Smith, 1999). Some of these feelings can be attributed to fear of the unknown and anticipatory anxiety (Davies et al., 1994; Gray and Smith, 1999). What you may not realise is that these feelings are perfectly natural, given the fact that you are about to embark on one of the biggest aspects of your pre-registration education. In fact, Kelly et al. (2007) say that you should expect to feel unsure of how to act and what to do, even if you have practised skills in a previous area.

Case study

Audrey recalls her first practice experience.

I remember the weekend before my first practice week I was just so nervous. It wasn't that I didn't want to go; in fact, I'd been desperate to get out in practice and start to see some real patients. I remember feeling really nervous, which was just awful because, the night before, I barely slept and couldn't eat at all on the morning I went. I actually felt physically sick. Looking back I realised that this was normal, it just showed how much I cared about what I was doing. Over time it's been easier to go to new practice areas as I'm better prepared and know what to do. You never stop feeling nervous, though, because practice is such a challenge, but it's also the best part of the course by a mile.

For obvious reasons, your very first practice experience is likely to be quite daunting, but most students continue to feel nervous prior to all their practice experiences. There will be new people to meet, a new environment to discover and a new set of learning objectives to achieve, so it is very important to acknowledge that, every time you embark on a practice learning experience, you will need to spend some time preparing for the occasion. If you do take responsibility and plan for what you can control about your learning experiences, fear of the unknown can be significantly reduced.

Why can't I just turn up for my practice experience?

It is sometimes difficult to understand why you need to prepare for all your practice experiences, especially if you have some prior experience to rely on. Spending time on preparation may even seem irrelevant when compared to all the other pressures of your training. It may also be tempting to skip your practice preparation if it is not included as an essential part of your coursework. When the pressures of theoretical work and exams are looming, practice preparation may just seem to be too much effort. Therefore, in order to put the whole issue of practice preparation into perspective, it is important to understand the impact preparation has on your learning experience as a whole.

> ## Scenario
>
> *Imagine you are about to go on a holiday to a country you have never visited. What type of preparation would you make before you left? You would probably spend considerable time organising your travel arrangements and ensuring you had accommodation arranged ahead of time. You may even 'Google' the destination, looking up important details such as nearby attractions or transport links. The reason you do this is to ensure you have an enjoyable time and make the most of the experience. If you didn't prepare you would possibly encounter many problems or miss out on many experiences. If you know what to take, you will avoid being at a loss or wasting time when you are there.*
>
> *Preparing for your practice learning experience has many similarities to planning for a trip to an unknown destination. You will need to consider issues such as travel, what to expect while you are there and the types of experiences that will be available.*

Be prepared

Being prepared for an event can prevent problems and reduce overall anxiety. The simple fact is that, if you put some time and effort into preparing for practice properly, this will pay dividends when you get there. If you don't prepare for your practice learning experiences, you will ultimately encounter problems and deny yourself the best and most valuable learning opportunities. The good news is that there are many things you can do to improve the experiences that you have in practice before you even get there. However, you will need to accept that you are responsible for your own practice preparation. Either you decide to do it or you don't. No one can prepare you for your experience apart from you.

Planning for learning success

Before you even contemplate setting foot in any practice area, you will need to plan for how you are going to learn. Some students make the big mistake of thinking that learning will just naturally happen once they turn up in practice. Kelly et al. (2007) term this a 'doing' attitude, where students rush into a practice experience with a big list of what they need to 'do', rather than what they need to 'learn'. In this case, many students will return from practice saying that they didn't learn anything (Elcock, 2006). This attitude can also result in a student feeling as if they are being used as an extra pair of hands, rather than being treated as a learner.

It is vitally important, therefore, that you enter the practice environment with an understanding of what you need to learn while you are there, and how you plan to do it. This will assist you to remain focused on these objectives from the very beginning. Elcock et al. (2007) argue that it is all too easy for mentors to mistake your participation in practice as a contribution to their work rather than your learning opportunity. This is far from the ideal situation, and it is easy to want to blame your mentor for this. However, if you think about it logically, you will realise that your mentor is not entirely responsible for your learning. Unless you know why you are there and what you should be doing, your mentor may just accept a situation in which you are helping to get the work done (Elcock, 2006).

Planning your learning outcomes

You must, therefore, enter your practice experience with a mindset as a 'learner' rather than a 'doer'. This means that you will need to review all your learning outcomes prior to your practice experience and start planning for how you will achieve these. The earlier you start preparing, the better; and leaving your preparation until the night before is hardly ideal.

Therefore, before your practice experience commences you should review your learning outcomes and draw up a list of everything you need to learn while you are there (Elcock, 2006). Not only will this help to keep you focused on what you need to learn, but it will make a great first impression when you meet your mentor. It will also help to clarify with your mentor that you are there to learn through doing, not just there to *do*.

Learning outcomes and learning opportunities

The first step is to start matching up your learning outcomes with learning opportunities – actually quite a simple process. Begin by making a list of the different learning outcomes you will be required to achieve during the practice experience. Once you have formulated your list, you can then start to plan the types of activities that may be available to you that match up with each learning opportunity. In other words, a list of *how* you plan to achieve the *what*.

Activity 3.2 — *Decision-making*

The aim of this activity is to improve your awareness of potential learning opportunities in practice. The table below provides an opportunity for you to make some decisions regarding the types of learning opportunities that would support your practice learning outcomes. There is one example learning outcome provided to get you started. Use the blank boxes to draw up your own list, making links between *what* you need to do and *how* you plan to do it. You may like to refer to a previous or current practice assessment booklet to make this activity realistic and relevant to your own experiences.

Learning outcome (What)	Learning opportunity (How)
Demonstrates appropriate verbal communication strategies when communicating with patients and members of the multidisciplinary team.	• Handover of patients • Answering the telephone • Participating in case conferences

continued overleaf . . .

continued . . .

Learning outcome (What)	Learning opportunity (How)

As this activity is based on your own observation, there is no outline answer at the end of the chapter.

Planning through using resources

There may be a number of resources available to you to help with planning your learning opportunities. For example, your university may have information about practice areas online and, if so, you will have been provided with information on how to access the required websites during your programme. If this resource is available to you, it is to your advantage to look at any practice information and complete any suggested preparation. Online resources often provide additional information to help with planning your learning experiences and what you can expect while you are there. They can be updated more frequently than printed material and, as a result, are a valuable source of information. Have a look at the learning outcomes and opportunities that you matched in Activity 3.2. There may well be very detailed information regarding the learning opportunities that will be available for each stage of your practice learning experiences. If this is the case, take full advantage of this information as it will give you a head start for each practice experience.

It is also likely that you will have been provided with suggested readings or activities to complete prior to undertaking your practice experience. In addition, you may be required to complete preparatory work in your assessment document before the practice experience begins. These may be e-learning activities, or presented to you in the form of classroom discussion or a workbook. You may even find that practice preparation forms part of your personal development portfolio, and there are specific requirements related to this. These may be in the form of reflections or activities, perhaps within a folder or online e-portfolio. It is quite possible that some of this work may be self-directed in nature and not directly linked to your assessment criteria. If this is the case, the temptation not to engage with preparatory work can be quite high.

It is common for students to dedicate the majority of their time to activities for which there are marks to be earned. It may also be difficult for you to see the relevance of the suggested readings to your next practice experience (Wilkinson et al., 1998). However, specific practice preparation is there to assist you in gaining independence in your practice learning. The more independent you are, the more you will enjoy your practice experience, as you will be given greater responsibility and have more opportunities to participate in learning experiences (Lofmark and Wikblad, 2001). If there is specific practice preparation recommended to you, you should definitely undertake this. If you fail to prepare adequately for practice you will be compromising your own learning experience.

Understanding where you are going

It is really important that you understand the nature of the practice area to which you will be going for your learning experience. Turning up on your first day without knowing about the practice area is a major mistake, and is actually quite insulting to the staff who work there. It will be noted that you have not taken the time to undertake preparatory research, as this will be reflected in the questions that you ask (Sharples, 2007a). Not only will the lack of preparation impact on your learning experience, but your mentor may interpret this as a lack of interest in their practice area. Inadequate preparation may result in a negative first impression of you and make it more difficult for you to fit into the practice environment (Fitzpatrick et al., 1996). Once again, there may be websites that you can access with this sort of information, and your university may have specific practice information available for you to access.

Case study

A mentor speaks about the frustration of having a student come into the practice area without making an effort to prepare.

We had this student a few months ago who just turned up on his first day and right from the start it was obvious he didn't have a clue what we do here. We're an orthopaedic ward, and he just stood there looking blank and it was very obvious he didn't know what the word 'orthopaedic' meant. He may as well have hung a big sign around his neck that said, 'I don't want to be here', as far as I was concerned. It was just so frustrating, for him and for us, because we just don't have time to spend hours explaining the basics that students should already know. If he had put the effort into us, we would have put the effort into him. In the end it took him about two weeks to catch on to what there was to learn and, by that time, he'd missed out on so much the whole thing was a bit of a waste really.

Planning a visit

In most cases you will find it useful to arrange a visit to your practice area as part of your preparation. It is never a good idea to turn up unannounced, so make a phone call or email to find out if a visit is suitable, and to arrange a good day and time. You may have an opportunity to meet key staff before your practice experience starts and familiarise yourself with the layout of the practice area (Sharples, 2007a). This is also a great way to introduce yourself to your mentor. All of this can help to reduce your pre-practice anxiety. Such a visit can also be a good way to plan for the learning opportunities available to you, as you may be able to ask more questions about the specialty. If your approach is right, it can also make a great first impression, as you will come across as keen, eager and prepared to learn.

Practical planning

Plan your travel

Obviously, you want to create the very best first impression when you turn up to practice on the first day, and arriving on time in the correct location is one of the best ways to do this. One of the easiest and least complicated aspects of preparing for a practice experience is planning how you will travel to and from your practice area. This may seem a little obvious, but often students have been caught out by this aspect, even those who have prepared thoroughly in other ways. If you have prepared for this, you will have more time to devote to learning and less to worrying about being late. Keep in mind also that your practice experience could involve travelling to a variety of locations and you may be expected to visit a number of different locations throughout the practice time. Not only should you prepare for how to get to your practice areas but also for how to get home. Depending on your circumstances, you may need to consider issues such as public transport links or parking facilities.

Top tips for planning travel

- Use a map to plan your journey to avoid getting lost and carry the map with you.
- If you are using public transport, check travel times for all your different shifts.
- Have a contingency plan for weekends and public holidays as your travel time may be longer or shorter than usual.
- If you are planning on driving or cycling, find out where you can park your car or bike safely for the duration of the shift.
- Find out the cost of parking meters and carry change if necessary.
- Consider a 'trial run' well in advance of your first day so you know what to expect during the journey and when you arrive.
- Use the resources your university has for planning journeys to practice areas, or online journey planners.
- Add some additional time to your planned journey to allow for last-minute problems, for example traffic delays.
- Don't forget to plan the journey home, as well as your journey to the practice area.

Life outside practice

On every practice experience that you undertake, you will need to consider how you are going to cope with and manage your life outside. Once again, you may be able to predict some events and to plan before practice how to manage these situations when they arise.

Shift work

Without any doubt, your practice experience will impact significantly on your home and family life. Shift work and the requirement for you to be directly or indirectly supervised at all times by your mentor will result in the need for you to do unsocial hours that may not fit in with current childcare arrangements or with social or work commitments. Unfortunately, some students make the mistake of thinking that, once they have informed the practice area of their special circumstances, adjustments will be made to their off-duty hours to accommodate their needs (Sharples, 2006). This is not the case and you should certainly not expect it. It is essential, therefore, that you make adequate arrangements before your practice experience commences so that your personal life does not impact on your availability for practice. The NMC makes your position, and your mentor's, very clear on this issue: *Whilst giving direct care in the practice setting at least 40 per cent of a student's time must be spent being supervised (directly or indirectly) by a mentor* (2008, p30).

The meaning of this directive is very clear. Every time you are involved in direct patient care during your practice experiences, a mentor is required to supervise you. Therefore, the onus is on you to be available to fit in with your mentor's rota and this leaves very limited options for negotiating your own shift pattern. Combine this directive with the NMC requirement that students must be exposed to the full range of 24-hour/7 days a week care in relation to practice experience (NMC, 2010) and it becomes very clear that very few adjustments will be made for your personal circumstances. You will need to plan for how to cope with this prior to your practice experiences.

Part-time work

Many students find that the difficulty of juggling part-time work commitments around practice experiences causes them considerable stress. As a result of the NMC regulations, it is impossible to have any sort of fixed work commitment as, sooner or later, it will clash with your practice experience. While there is no problem with you having a job while you are undertaking your nursing course, any employment must be flexible around your practice experiences, not the other way round. The same goes for the theory part of the programme. In other words, you will need to arrange your life to meet the requirements of the nursing programme; the programme cannot be altered to suit you. For this reason, your best option for part-time work would be casual employment, perhaps as part of a nursing bank or agency.

Smoking

If you are a smoker, you will need to plan for how to cope with this during your practice experiences. The days of smoking in tearooms and designated smoking areas are long gone, so a quick cigarette break while in practice is out of the question. Remember that the NHS has now gone smoke free, meaning that there are no smoking areas within NHS grounds. Very often this applies not only to buildings but also to outside perimeter areas. If you have to go some distance to find a suitable outdoor area in which to smoke, this will not be viable during your practice experience. Leaving the practice area for a cigarette will be viewed as unprofessional and will also have a negative impact on your learning opportunities (Elcock, 2007). Your options are to consider giving up smoking prior to your practice experience, or to plan for some type of nicotine replacement that will curb your cravings. Whatever you decide to do is up to you; the most important thing is that you do have a plan of how to cope. This may seem trivial; however, for many students this can affect their enjoyment and commitment to practice.

Sickness and absences

Obviously, some events are unpredictable and cannot always be specifically planned for. However, you can plan ahead for what you will do when unpredictable events do occur. For example, sickness and burst water pipes can all happen with very little warning, but may result in you being unable to attend practice. You will therefore need to have contact details available of relevant people whom you may need to inform if you cannot attend your practice area. Extended periods of absence will have an impact on your learning opportunities, so you should make yourself aware of relevant policies before the practice experience commences. At the very least, you should review your student policy on sickness and absence, as this will provide information on what to do and whom to contact, and check the policy on make-up time, to provide support for you should you need it.

Final preparation

Before you embark on your practice experience, the final step is to make sure absolutely everything you need to do and plan for is in order. Remember that, the more you plan, the less likely it is that you will encounter unpredictable events.

Activity 3.3	*Reflection*

Use this checklist to ensure that you really are prepared for all aspects of your practice experience. Put a tick next to each of the elements that applies to you.

I know where I am going for my practice learning experiences.	
I have organised my travel arrangements.	
I have reviewed my learning outcomes.	
I have matched my learning outcomes with learning opportunities.	
I have arranged a pre-practice visit.	
I have the contact numbers and details of where I am going.	
I have done the preparation work recommended to me.	
I have looked at the website for practice area information (if available).	
I know exactly where to go and whom to ask for when I get there.	
I am available for the full range of shifts that I might be required to do.	

continued opposite . . .

continued . . .

I have reviewed my university policies on sickness and make-up time.	
I have the contact details of lecturers I may need to call while in practice.	
I know whom to contact if I cannot attend practice.	
I have planned how to cope with my nicotine cravings (if required).	
I have a uniform or appropriate clothes as required.	
I have completed the relevant sections of my practice assessment document.	

As this activity is for your own reflection, there is no outline answer at the end of the chapter.

Use this opportunity to reflect on the answers you gave for Activity 3.1. What aspects of practice experience were you concerned about when we began this chapter? If you are able to tick each box confidently in the checklist in Activity 3.3, it is very likely that your original fears have been well and truly dealt with. In most cases, your original fears were related to the unknown, and preparation for practice experiences allows you to confront and deal with this.

If you still have some concerns regarding your practice preparation, it is important that you deal with these issues. Failing to solve a problem does not make it go away; it simply means that your problem will be deferred to a later date when it is likely to cause you considerable stress and anxiety. Now is the time to be honest regarding potential obstacles that may impact on your practice experience. You will need to consider your options for resolving the problem, either yourself or by discussing solutions with partners, friends or university staff.

Case study

Cherry is a first-year student whose relationship ended the week before her practice experience. She had hoped that her boyfriend would be available to assist with childcare, but since the break-up he has refused to care for his son. Cherry decides to attend her practice experience without discussing her situation with her programme leader; she reasons that the practice area will support her request for Monday to Friday morning shifts. The practice area can accommodate no such request; all mentors are rostered on rotating shifts and Cherry's request does not support the Standards to Support Learning and Assessment in Practice (NMC, 2008b). Cherry has no alternative but to take sick leave for all afternoon, night and weekend shifts. At the end of the practice experience, Cherry has accrued over 150 hours of sick leave. As this time cannot be made up, Cherry finds herself withdrawn from the programme. If Cherry had discussed her predicament with her programme leader, it may have been possible for her to transfer to a Monday to Friday practice area for a short period of time to allow alternative childcare to be found.

Problems and solutions

It may be that, despite working through the checklist, you still have some areas of concern that have not been resolved. If this is the case, you must resolve these issues before your practice experience begins. You will need to identify exactly what your concerns are in order to find a solution. Identifying any likely problems and what you can actively do about these issues will help you to feel more in control of your practice experience and more confident regarding your performance as a whole.

Activity 3.4 · Critical thinking

Use the following table to write down any concerns you may have regarding your upcoming practice experience. Next to each problem write down what you feel the solution might be. Try to be as systematic as possible as problems are best dealt with step by step. Once you have decided upon a possible solution it is up to you to make this happen.

Pre-practice concerns	Solutions

An outline of some example concerns and solutions is given at the end of the chapter.

Chapter summary

In this chapter we have discussed the importance of preparing for practice experiences and how thorough preparation can improve your overall learning opportunities. Understanding what, how and when to prepare for your practice experience is vital in terms of reducing your anxiety and making the most of all learning opportunities that may come your way. The choice regarding how much or little you do in terms of your practice preparation is down to you, and it will require a certain amount of self-direction and intrinsic motivation. However, while there will be some effort required, it will not go to waste and, ultimately, you will be the one to reap the rewards.

Activities: Brief outline answers

Activity 3.4 Pre-practice concerns and solutions (page 48)

This activity required you to think through some possible concerns you may have prior to your practice experience and consider the solutions. Some examples of genuine student problems and their solutions are given below.

Concern – I've just moved from Ireland to London and am not sure how to travel to all my practice areas as I don't know London at all.

Solution – The Transport for London website has a journey planner function that allows you to find a range of alternative routes by using postcodes. As the postcodes for all my practice areas are on the practice website, I can find out how to travel to any location.

Concern – My sister died last year and I'm still finding it hard to cope. I'm really worried about having to care for patients with cancer as this reminds me of my sister.

Solution – My university has a free counselling service for students. I can book in and talk to someone neutral about my feelings and how to cope with caring for cancer patients.

Further reading

Elcock, K (2006) Wake up and learn. *Nursing Standard*, 20(49): 61.

This is a short article that provides insight into student experiences in practice.

Useful websites

www.rcn.org.uk/__data/assets/pdf_file/0011/78545/001815.pdf

This toolkit, entitled 'Helping students get the most from their practice placements', provides an overview of the student role and responsibilities while on practice experience. There is a small section on student responsibility in relation to practice preparation.

Chapter 4
Working with my mentor

NMC Standards for Pre-registration Nursing Education

This chapter will address the following competencies:

Domain 1: Professional values

5. All nurses must fully understand the nurse's various roles, responsibilities and functions, and adapt their practice to meet the changing needs of people, groups, communities and populations.

8. All nurses must practice independently, recognising the limits of their competence and knowledge. They must reflect on these limits and seek advice from, or refer to, other professionals where necessary.

Domain 2: Communication and interpersonal skills

1. All nurses must build partnerships and therapeutic relationships through safe, effective and non-discriminatory communication. They must take account of individual differences, capabilities and needs.

Domain 4: Leadership, management and team working

3. All nurses must be self aware and recognise how their own values, principles and assumptions might affect their practice. They must maintain their own personal and professional development, learning from experience, through supervision, feedback, reflection and evaluation.

NMC Essential Skills Clusters

This chapter will address the following ESCs:

Cluster: Care, compassion and communication

7. People can trust the newly registered graduate nurse to protect and keep as confidential all information relating to them.

Cluster: Organisational aspects of care

10. People can trust the newly registered graduate nurse to deliver nursing interventions and evaluate their effectiveness against the agreed assessment and care plan.

19. People can trust the newly registered graduate nurse to work to prevent and resolve conflict and maintain a safe environment.

Introduction: learning in practice

In Chapter 2 we dealt with the primary expectations of you as an adult learner. However, it is also likely that you will have some expectations related to the type of support you should receive during your practice experience. Obviously, learning is a two-way process and, in many ways, your learning will be related to and directly affected by the quality of the learning environment in which you undertake your practice experience.

The aim of this chapter is to help you understand the nature of the practice environment, the role of your **mentor** and the factors related to practice support. We will start by considering your current understanding of how your role in practice fits with the mentor's role. Next, we will examine the standards the NMC expects of mentors and also the type and nature of support your university is required to provide for you in practice. The role of the mentor will then be looked at in some detail, as well as your mentor's accountability. The additional support mentors can access is then covered, and the chapter ends by looking at the role of sign-off mentors.

Expectations of practice learning

Before you can even begin to learn in practice, you will need to have a very clear understanding of what your role is in practice and how this fits with your mentor's role. The student grapevine is notorious for turning myths into what seem like facts, so for this reason it is very likely that you may have heard stories or information about practice learning that are untrue and therefore incorrect. If this is the case, your expectations of your mentor in relation to practice learning will also be incorrect. False assumptions tend to lead to false conclusions. If you attend your practice area with incorrect expectations and false assumptions, the consequence can be an unfulfilling and negative experience. The starting point, therefore, is to begin by looking at the real facts regarding practice experiences, and hopefully dispel once and for all some common myths along the way.

Activity 4.1   *Reflection*

No doubt you will have some beliefs about your practice experience and what you can expect from your mentor. Use the space below to finish the sentence about the expectations you have in relation to your mentor. List as many things as you can that you feel your mentor should provide for you during your practice experience.

I expect that, during my practice experience, my mentor will . . .

For the time being you don't have to do anything with this list. However, from time to time during this chapter you will be asked to come back and refer to your list to remind yourself of your expectations.

As this activity is for your own reflection, there is no outline answer at the end of the chapter.

NMC standards regarding practice support

The list you have made in Activity 4.1 will contain the support you expect to receive from your mentor. What you may not realise is that the NMC has already decided on the level of support mentors are required to provide for you. The NMC has set very clear guidelines regarding this support, and these guidelines are listed in the *Standards to Support Learning and Assessment in Practice* (NMC, 2008b). These standards were first published in August 2006 and came into force on 1 September 2007. In July 2008 the standards were updated, and these are the guidelines that your mentor is expected to follow. Importantly for you, one section of these NMC standards states that you must be provided with appropriate support from your university and also the practice area while you undertake practice experiences. Thus, while you may have your own personal expectations, it is actually the NMC that sets the criteria and expectations for your support and assessment during your learning experience.

University support

You will already be aware that practice learning equates to 50 per cent of your total training, so 2,300 hours of your pre-registration programme will be spent in practice. The NMC makes it very clear to your university that students should be supported in both academic and practice learning environments (NMC, 2010). In order to ensure that you are adequately supported in practice, your university is required to audit the practice learning environment to identify the number and nature of students that may be effectively supported (NMC, 2010). This is to ensure that the practice area where you undertake your experience is the right sort of environment for your learning needs. These reviews are carried out either annually or biannually and your university is required to submit these reviews to the NMC when quality inspections are undertaken. There are many factors that are taken into consideration when deciding on whether a practice area can and should support students during their practice experiences, and your university and the area will make these decisions in partnership.

The role of a mentor

Your day-to-day support during practice experiences is undertaken by a mentor. Therefore, it is very important that we now take the time to look at the specifics of a mentor's role and responsibility in far more detail, paying particular attention, in this section, to how your mentor should fulfil their role.

Who is a mentor?

Let us start by defining who a mentor is, based on the NMC definition:

> *An NMC mentor is a registrant who, following successful completion of an NMC approved mentor preparation programme, has achieved the knowledge, skills and competence required to meet the defined outcomes.*
> (NMC, 2008b, p19)

This means that your mentor must have completed and passed an NMC-approved mentorship course in order to gain a mentorship qualification. From this point on, a mentor is professionally bound to adhere to the *Standards to Support Learning and Assessment in Practice* (NMC, 2008b).

Mentor support

Once qualified, the NMC requires mentors to support learning in practice in a variety of different ways. These can be found in the above-mentioned standards (NMC, 2008b) and have been summarised as follows.

- To provide support and guidance to students when learning new skills or applying new knowledge.
- To act as a resource to the student to facilitate learning and professional growth.
- To directly manage a student's learning in practice to ensure public protection.
- To directly observe a student's practice, or use indirect observation where appropriate, in order to ensure that NMC-defined outcomes and competencies are met.

Therefore, as the name would suggest, your mentor's role according to the NMC standards is to support your learning and to support your assessment. We will look at each of these aspects in turn.

Support of learning in practice

The NMC makes it very clear that your mentor is required to coordinate appropriate learning experiences for you during your practice. This is quite a substantial role and involves both of you working together in partnership to ensure that you are provided with realistic and appropriate experiences. Both you and your mentor will need to have a very good understanding of your learning goals in order to choose and maximise the best range of learning experiences.

Activity 4.2   *Reflection*

Take the opportunity now to reflect on the list you created in Activity 4.1 regarding the expectations of your mentor.

- Are any of your expectations focused on the facilitation of your learning?
- Have you mentioned anything that suggests that your mentor will be supportive of your learning?
- Based on the notes you wrote for Activity 4.1, are your expectations accurate and realistic, regarding the *Standards to Support Learning and Assessment in Practice* (NMC, 2008b)?

As this activity is for your own reflection, there is no outline answer at the end of the chapter.

If your previous expectations of your mentor are very different from what you now understand about their role, take some time now to reflect on your answers to Activity 4.2. Consider why this may be the case. Have you relied on other students to advise you on the role of the mentor, or have you made assumptions based on your own feelings? Unless your source of information regarding the role of your mentor is from a reliable source, it is likely that the information you have will be incorrect. For factual information you could refer to either the *Standards to Support Learning and Assessment in Practice* (NMC, 2008b) or university information regarding your mentor's role. Very often this will be preprinted for you in your practice assessment document.

One of the more common misconceptions held by students is that your mentor will act as a teacher during your practice experience. If so, then take note that this is inaccurate and unrealistic. It is the type of myth that is assumed by students to be fact. However, the NMC makes it very clear that your mentor is not required to be your teacher. Some students find this a very difficult concept to grasp, and have an expectation that their mentor will allocate time to undertake 'teaching'. On the contrary, it is expected that, as an adult learner, you will be more inclined to engage with facilitation of learning experiences rather than relying on didactic teaching. We will have the opportunity to explore this further in Chapters 5 and 6, where we will discuss self-regulated learning and **experiential learning**. In the meantime, it is worth having a look at the accountability and responsibility of mentors within the *Standards to Support Learning and Assessment in Practice* (NMC, 2008b).

Accountability and responsibility of mentors

- *Organising and coordinating student learning activities in practice.*
- *Supervising students in learning situations and providing them with constructive feedback on their achievements.*
- *Setting and monitoring achievement of realistic learning objectives.*
- *Assessing total performance – including knowledge, skills, attitudes and behaviours.*
- *Providing evidence . . . of student achievement or lack of achievement.*
- *Liaising with others . . . to provide feedback, identify any concerns . . . and agree action as appropriate.*

(NMC, 2008b)

Facilitation of learning

It is very clear from this list that the NMC requires your mentor to be focused on the facilitation of your learning, rather than teaching. In fact, 'teaching' is not mentioned at all. This concept fits in very neatly with the notion of an adult learner that we dealt with in Chapter 2. Remember that, as an adult learner, it will be expected that you will take mutual responsibility for your learning, rather than expect it to be done for you. You will have an opportunity to discover ways in which you and your mentor will be engaging with learning experiences described in Chapter 6.

Case study

A mentor speaks about their experience of facilitating student learning.

I actually love mentoring students. It's really rewarding when you have a student who is just so keen to learn everything they can, and you're able to see them becoming more confident as they develop their skills with the patients. It keeps me on my toes as well, especially when we discuss a patient's care plan or treatment. The last student I mentored asked me something about a new procedure I'd never heard of and that was great; we ended up learning something new together.

That's why I find it so hard when a student just isn't interested in learning. Some students just seem to hang around, as if they're waiting for me to teach them something. We just have so many demands on our time now that it's not possible to do separate student teaching. If I could give students one piece of advice it would be to know what it is they want to learn and not expect their mentor to work it out for them. That's why my last student had such a great practice experience; he just knew what he wanted to do and it made all the difference. In the first week he asked if it would be OK for him to get his own patient caseload every day and for me to give him feedback at the end of the shift. I said to him 'brilliant – you go for it.' I really respected the fact that he came to me with what he wanted and didn't want to waste his time.

The main point is that you should attend your practice experience with a very clear understanding of what it is you would like to learn and the types of experiences you would like to engage with in order to fulfil your learning outcomes. The NMC then requires your mentor to coordinate and facilitate appropriate learning opportunities according to your individual needs.

Learning takes place through the feedback you receive. This means that the real driver of your learning is you. If you undertake a practice experience without a clear understanding of your learning objectives, your mentor will have nothing to facilitate. The risk is that, with no clear objectives, you may be seen as an extra pair of hands rather than as a learner (Johnson and Preston, 2001).

Case study

Elizabeth is undertaking a practice experience in a children's day-care unit. By the second week, several mentors have noticed that Elizabeth seems to lack motivation and, on a number of occasions, she has been late back from her lunch break. She has been offered opportunities to assess children coming into the unit and to help develop treatment plans, but she seems reluctant to involve herself and sits down regularly at the desk. When Elizabeth attends the daily planning meeting she does not ask to be allocated her own patients, and prefers to shadow her mentor throughout the shift. Elizabeth's mentor decides to question her regarding her motivation as she is clearly unhappy. Elizabeth explains that she is unhappy because she feels she is not learning anything on the practice experience.

Her mentor cannot understand this comment and reminds Elizabeth that she has been offered responsibility every day for her own patients: to help admit them into the unit, plan, manage and deliver care, and organise discharges throughout the day. 'Oh I know,' says Elizabeth, 'but I'm not learning – no one is teaching me anything.'

Support of assessment in practice

The second role that your mentor must fulfil during your practice experience is to assess your competence. When you arrive in practice you will already have been provided with a set of learning outcomes. It is your mentor's job to assess you on these outcomes during your practice experience. The learning opportunities that you engage with during your practice will provide your mentor with an opportunity to observe your practice and make a judgement about your competence. Your mentor is required by the NMC to assess your total performance in order to determine competence (NMC, 2008b).

Have a look at Figure 4.1. This represents the three aspects of competence that you will be assessed on for each of your learning outcomes. You will note that all aspects of competence are of equal importance, so your knowledge, for example, is no less or more important than your attitude or skill. It is very important that you understand that your competence will be judged not just on what you can do (skills; also known as psychomotor skills), but also on what you know (knowledge; also known as cognitive skills) and the way you act (attitude; also known as affective

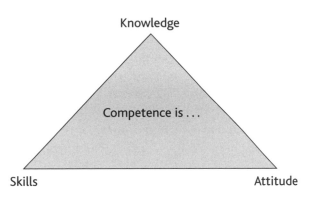

Figure 4.1: What is competence?

skills). Just as we discussed in Chapter 1, you must prove to your mentor that you are a 'knowledgeable doer'.

How competent do I need to be?

The competence level that you will be expected to meet has been set by the NMC and outlined within the *Standards for Pre-registration Nursing Education* (NMC, 2010). We first looked at the contents of this document when examining the design of your pre-registration curriculum in Chapter 1 and also in the Introduction to this book, so it may be worth referring back to these to refresh your memory. The fact is that all your learning outcomes will be related to the competency level expected of you at each stage of your nursing programme. It should come as no surprise, therefore, that both of these documents also contain information related to your practice assessment and the role of your mentor. In fact, no matter what stage of the programme you are on, your mentor will be required to assess you against NMC standards, whether this is to progress on your course or to qualify as a nurse.

Mentor accountability and responsibility

Your mentor is accountable and responsible to the NMC for all the assessment decisions they make about you. The following statement in the *Standards to Support Learning and Assessment in Practice* makes this very clear:

> *Mentors will have been prepared to assess student performance in practice and will be accountable for their decisions to pass, refer or fail a student.*
> (NMC, 2008b, p32)

The NMC provides each university with very clear guidelines on the structure and nature of your practice assessment. In turn, your university will provide you with a practice assessment document that is based on these guidelines. Your mentor is professionally obligated to follow this assessment process, as the NMC will hold them accountable for the assessment decision they make about you. The assessment process that your mentor is required to follow means that they must provide evidence of your achievement or lack of achievement during your practice experiences.

Feedback on competence

Typically, the evidence of your competence that your mentor must provide will be in the form of documented notes within your practice assessment document or practice portfolio, and verbal feedback throughout your practice learning experience. This is to ensure that you are kept well informed of your progress. However, the feedback is not just for your benefit. At the end of your practice experience, the NMC requires your mentor to document your progress within an 'ongoing achievement record'. This is to allow comments and feedback from your mentor to be passed on to your next practice area in order to enable your next mentor to make judgements on your progress (NMC, 2008b).

The feedback you receive, both written and verbal, is an essential aspect of your learning experience, so we will deal with this subject in far more depth later in this book. For the time being, it is important to understand that the provision of feedback is not optional, and the NMC requires your mentor to do this because it is fundamental to your learning. The documentation that your mentor provides within your assessment document also furnishes evidence that your assessment has been undertaken fairly, accurately and according to assessment guidelines. Without such documentation there is no proof that your assessment has met the required standards set by the NMC.

Additional practice support

If your mentor has concerns about your progress during a practice experience, the NMC requires them to seek help. Some students find this particular aspect of the mentor role very difficult to understand and this can lead to them feeling that they have been betrayed by their mentor. However, it is very important to understand that your mentor is not your friend, but your assessor. This is not to say that your mentor should not be friendly; but their role is functional and does not have the same features, functions or attributes as a friendship.

From the time your practice experience begins, your mentor is under significant pressure to make an accurate and objective assessment decision regarding your competence. They just cannot afford to get this wrong. If they require help in their mentoring role, the NMC makes it very clear that they should ask for it.

Scenario

Georgiana has just passed her driving test and decides to buy her first car. She spends a whole weekend looking through magazines, searching the internet and walking around car dealerships. By the end of the weekend she has some idea about the best car to buy, but decides to get some help from others before making her final decision. Her best friend, Dorothy, has driven a similar model before and is able to share her experiences. Her grandfather, Keith, is a retired mechanic and offers to go with Georgiana on another test drive. Her brother, Michael, has had recent experience buying his own car and gives her some advice regarding finance options. After making use of all this advice and support Georgiana is far more confident about her decision and becomes the proud owner of her first car.

The point of the above scenario is that, when important decisions need to be made, it is good practice to share your dilemma with someone else who can offer a different perspective and may be able to suggest alternatives that have not yet occurred to you. The value of someone else's opinion when faced with a difficult problem is often invaluable. The same can be said for mentors who are concerned about your progress.

Support for mentors

The support your mentor may access can include other mentors, practice teachers, practice facilitators or link tutors from your university. They may ask for assistance with the facilitation of your learning experiences, action planning or assessment strategies (NMC, 2008b). Your mentor can also ask that other members of the teaching and healthcare team contribute to your learning and assessment in practice; however, they alone will be accountable and responsible for undertaking the summative assessment of your learning outcomes (NMC, 2004). It is reasonable, therefore, to expect that a range of people may be involved with the facilitation of your learning, discussing your progress and assessment of your competence.

Activity 4.3   *Reflection*

Once again, reflect on the expectations you had of a mentor at the beginning of this chapter.

- Think about the expectations you had of your mentor in relation to assessment, learning and feedback.
- How have your expectations changed?

Based on what you have learned in this chapter, you may like to use the space below to summarise your new expectations.

By writing these down you will be able to clarify the expectations you have for your mentor and also what their expectations will be of you.

- Now that you have a clearer understanding of the role of your mentor during your practice experiences, how will this change your approach to your next practice event?
- How will you check that your expectations remain accurate, especially as you move through future practice experiences?

As this activity is for your own reflection, there is no outline answer at the end of the chapter.

Sign-off mentors

By now you should have a very clear understanding of your mentor's role in relation to your practice learning. However, in order to safeguard the health and well-being of the public, the NMC must be assured that, at the end of your programme, you have been assessed and signed off as capable of safe and effective practice (NMC, 2008). As a result, the NMC has decided that the mentor who makes the final decision regarding your competence for registration must fulfil additional criteria, and will be called a **sign-off mentor**.

How will the sign-off mentor role affect you?

It is very important to understand if and when the sign-off mentor role will affect you. If you began your pre-registration nurse training after 1 September 2007, you will need to be assessed on your final practice experience by a sign-off mentor. The practice period during which you will require a sign-off mentor will depend on the length of your course of study and the programme you are on, so you will be kept informed of this by your university. Needless to say, practice areas throughout the UK are constantly developing sign-off mentors in order to ensure that there are adequate mentors for all pre-registration nursing students on final practice experiences.

When you are being assessed during your final practice experience by a sign-off mentor, it is important to understand that the criteria for your assessment will not change, and neither will the criteria you will need to demonstrate in order to achieve competence. It will mean, however, that your mentor should be given protected time to provide feedback when undertaking their mentoring role, as this should be made possible under the mandatory time specification for sign-off mentors (Sharples, 2007b). Keep in mind, though, that, as the fundamental aspects of mentorship, facilitation of learning and assessment of competence remain unchanged, the sign-off mentor role will be an adjunct, rather than a change, to your final practice experience.

> ### Chapter summary
>
> The role of the mentor is very clearly defined within the *Standards to Support Learning and Assessment in Practice* (NMC, 2008b). In order to make the most of your learning opportunities during practice experiences, it is very important that you have clear and accurate expectations of your mentor. In this chapter we have looked at the role of the mentor in relation to both your learning experience and assessment of competence. The criterion for assessment of competence has been addressed, as has the professional obligation of a mentor in terms of written and verbal feedback. Additional support for mentors during a student's practice experience can promote objective assessment and, as such, is an NMC requirement to support learning and assessment.

Further reading

Elcock, K and Sharples, K (2011) *A Nurse's Survival Guide to Mentoring.* London: Elsevier.

This is a useful text that explains the role of the mentor and the mentoring process from the perspective of the mentor. It is a useful guide for understanding facilitation of learning from the perspective of the mentor.

Nursing and Midwifery Council (NMC) (2008) *Standards to Support Learning and Assessment in Practice: NMC standards for mentors, practice teachers and teachers.* London: NMC.

The NMC standard is quite a long document, but it does provide a comprehensive overview of the professional accountability and responsibility of mentors.

Useful websites

www.rcn.org.uk/search?queries_search_query=MENTOR+TOOLKIT

The RCN mentor toolkit can be downloaded from the RCN website. The toolkit offers tips and advice for mentors on facilitating your learning experiences during your practice learning experience.

Chapter 5
Planning my practice experience

Chapter aims

The aim of this chapter is for you understand how you can plan your learning experiences in practice.

After reading this chapter you will be able to:

- understand the link between planning learning and learning through experience;
- apply the principles of a learning cycle in order to plan your practice learning experiences;
- identify how you can use reflection to learn during practice experiences.

Introduction: learning to learn in practice

Every time you undertake a practice learning experience, you will have the chance to learn in, through and during a range of practice opportunities. The opportunities that you may encounter might be planned, foreseeable structured events, or random, coincidental and spontaneous. The nature of the event matters little, as all events, whether predictable or spontaneous, have one essential thing in common – they are all potential learning experiences.

Yet the opportunity to learn in practice does not automatically mean that learning will take place. Some students make the mistake of thinking that, once they are in practice, learning will just naturally happen. However, learning does not just happen; you will have to *make* it happen. First, you will need to develop the skills of an adult learner (Chapter 2) and, second, you will need to assume responsibility for your learning experiences. In addition, any barriers that may impact on your ability to learn must be dealt with, either by removing these barriers or reducing their impact so that you are free to learn.

Therefore, while there are opportunities to learn in practice, it is also important to seek out and use these opportunities. In this chapter we will discover how to do just that. The starting point will be to establish the types of practice experiences that may be developed into learning experiences. From this point, we will discuss how to use self-regulation to plan and structure learning, using Kolb's experiential learning cycle as an example. This will include an opportunity to see how planning for learning can be integrated into each stage of your practice learning experience, beginning with the initial interview and ending with the final interview. As well as exploring how you can learn by using a learning cycle, we will examine how to use reflection as a means of learning during and after practice experiences. The chapter will conclude by discussing how your learning experience can be designed to match with your individual learning style within a learning cycle.

Learning through practice experiences

The practice environment is a never-ending source of potential learning experiences that become more meaningful the more you participate (Andrews and Roberts, 2003). In fact, some experiences are guaranteed to occur every day. For example, if you are on a ward in a hospital, you can be certain that there will be medications administered to patients during the course of the shift. Likewise, if you are on a community practice learning experience in a day centre, you will have opportunities to communicate with service users. There will also be experiences available that cannot be planned for. For example, a patient you are caring for on a hospital ward may suddenly experience a drop in blood pressure and require urgent treatment. Or a client in a day centre may have a verbal argument with another client and you may need rapidly to diffuse a tense situation. In fact, virtually everything that takes place during your practice experience can be turned into an opportunity for you to learn.

The challenge is knowing how to turn your practice experiences into learning experiences. Unless you do this, your practice experiences will become a series of random events and learning opportunities will be wasted. A good starting point is for you to know how to identify the types of experiences, both planned and unplanned, that you may encounter in your practice area.

You could consider doing this as part of your preparation for practice as we discussed in Chapter 3. An essential starting point here is to ensure that you thoroughly understand the level of competency that will be expected of you throughout your pre-registration training. As the majority of your learning outcomes will be based directly on the competency statements set by the NMC, you should aim to become familiar with how your learning outcomes for each practice experience link with these statements.

It may be that planning for specific learning experiences is an important aspect of maintaining a personal development plan or practice portfolio. If you do not plan specific opportunities prior to the practice experience, you will need to undertake this prior to the initial interview with your mentor. If you have not planned any learning experiences, the initial interview could be a very limited discussion that is generalised rather than specific to your needs.

Remember also that the NMC expects you to keep a record of your learning experiences, identifying evidence to support achievement of NMC outcomes and competencies and where further support and supervision is required (NMC, 2008b). This record (often in the form of a portfolio) should be made available to your named mentor at the beginning of a new experience to enable discussion of strengths and areas for improvement.

Consider the practice experience

In planning your learning experiences it is very important that you make yourself aware of the variety of practice opportunities that you may encounter. The days of long 'practice placements' in just one area are slowly being phased out, so you cannot assume that you will be in one location for all of your practice weeks. The NMC has stopped using the term 'practice placement' and instead refers to 'practice learning opportunities' (NMC, 2010). This has allowed greater flexibility in the type of practice experience that may be provided. As long as you are exposed to learning experiences that will allow you to meet programme requirements, and as long as mentorship standards are maintained, your practice experience can take on any form that fits these criteria (NMC, 2010).

Examples of practice learning opportunities

Adult field

You may commence your practice experience in a surgical ward, learning about the care of patients before invasive procedures. You may then be given the opportunity to attend theatre over a number of days, gaining insight into the care of patients undergoing operations and the immediate recovery period. You may then return to your surgical ward where you focus on post-operative care and discharge planning, perhaps even participating in home visits. Throughout this practice experience your mentor in the surgical ward will monitor your progress and coordinate your learning experiences, including review of these experiences, providing feedback and ensuring you receive your initial, midpoint and final interviews.

Child field

You may commence your practice experience with the paediatric community team and gain experience in caring for children with long-term conditions such as asthma. You may then spend some time in a hospital children's ward, learning about the care of acutely sick children. The practice experience could also involve spending time with a school nurse, experiencing first-hand management issues for children with a range of chronic illnesses. Throughout this practice experience your mentor in the surgical ward will monitor your progress and coordinate your learning experiences, providing feedback and ensuring you receive your initial, midpoint and final interviews.

Learning disability field

You may commence your practice experience in a residential setting, learning about the care of adults with sensory disabilities. Your experience could include spending time with your clients in adult education, perhaps learning about the facilitation of reasonable adjustments under disability discrimination legislation. You may even have an opportunity to extend your learning experience by working with social workers and occupational therapists. Throughout this practice experience your mentor in the residential setting will monitor your progress and coordinate your learning experiences, providing feedback and ensuring you receive your initial, midpoint and final interviews.

Mental health field

You may commence your practice experience in an acute mental health unit, caring for clients with a wide range of mental health issues. Your learning experience could involve spending some time with community psychiatric nurses, attending home visits or perhaps supporting clients attending work interviews. Your learning experience could include spending time with practice nurses, learning about the assessment of clients' physical health needs. Throughout this practice experience your mentor in the mental health unit will monitor your progress and coordinate your learning experiences, providing feedback and ensuring you receive your initial, midpoint and final interviews.

Activity 5.1   *Critical thinking*

Use the grid to make a note of a few different types of experiences that could occur during your practice experience. Pay particular attention to whether the experiences are predictable or unpredictable. There is an example in each column to get you started. Ideally, you should do this prior to your initial interview.

Predictable experiences	Unpredictable experiences
Documenting in client notes	Making changes to a client's care plan following an MDT meeting

As this activity is based on your own reflection, there is no outline answer at the end of the chapter.

Take some time to consider the differences between the two lists you made in Activity 5.1. No doubt you found it quite difficult to identify unpredictable experiences. If you have very limited experience of a practice area before the experience commences, you may have a very clear understanding of the predictable learning experiences you will encounter, but only a limited perspective of other opportunities available to you. Additionally, if your practice experience involves moving through a number of different practice areas, you may initially find it quite challenging to know what learning opportunities will be available to you. Remember, though, that this state will change as you gain more experience in your learning environment. So your understanding of potential learning experiences will develop over time and should not be limited to your first impressions. We will address this concept again later in the chapter.

Predictable and unpredictable learning experiences

It should now be very clear that, while practice learning is all about experiences, it is actually impossible to predict a significant percentage of the experiences that you will encounter. This is especially true in the first days of your practice experiences. The paradox is that a great deal of your learning, and sometimes the best experiences, will take place as a result of unplanned, unexpected, random experiences.

The great news is that it is possible to learn through all experiences whether they are predictable or not. The key is having a plan of how to make the most of all your experiences, both predictable and unpredictable, to ensure that you are able to turn them into learning experiences. You may not be able to plan or predict what will take place in practice; however, you can plan for how you can learn from all experiences that come your way.

Learning through personal experience

Before we go any further, it is important to establish that people experience the same events in different ways. No doubt you have already been in a situation where your experience of an event was the exact opposite of someone else's. Boud et al. (1993) explain that this happens because the meaning of an experience is not a given, but is subject to interpretation.

Activity 5.2   *Critical thinking*

Take some time to consider the following statement:

> *When different learners are involved in the same event, their experience of it will be different and they will construct and reconstruct it differently. What learners bring to an event – their expectations, knowledge, attitude and emotions – will influence their interpretation of it and their own construction of what they experience. An event can influence a learner but only if the learner is predisposed to being influenced.*
> (Boud et al., 1993, p11)

Now think about a time in your life when you shared an experience with someone but had a different reaction. You may choose to relate this to a practice experience, or to something in your personal life.

*   Why do you think this happened?
*   What factors may have influenced your different reactions?

You may like to make some brief notes about the expectations, knowledge, attitude and emotions that influenced your interpretation of the event.

As this activity is based on your own observation, there is no outline answer at the end of the chapter.

Case study

Jenny and Isaac are pre-registration students in the learning disability field. A guest speaker comes to a tutorial session and speaks about deprivation of liberty legislation. Jenny is fascinated; she thinks the guest speaker is very interesting and, in particular, she appreciates his anecdotes and experiences from practice. She is disappointed when the session finishes after just one hour. Isaac found the session tedious and irrelevant.

continued overleaf . . .

continued . . . .

He thought the guest speaker rambled in the discussion without sticking to the key points and he felt the session could have been more beneficial if it had been limited to one hour.

When they discuss the tutorial the next day, Jenny and Isaac are surprised to find that they have had such different opinions. They realise that Jenny has enjoyed the session because her learning style is that of a theorist and she has a background in law. As a result, Jenny is naturally drawn to discussions that involve debate over legal concepts. Conversely, Isaac's learning style is that of a pragmatist and he prefers to be involved with applying legal principles in practice rather than talking about them or listening to other people discuss their experience. Isaac realises that he would have enjoyed the discussion much more if he had first experienced examples of the legislation being used by nurses in practice.

Making learning personal

What and how you learn from the experiences that you encounter in practice will be personal to you. The fact that you will be exposed to practice experiences does not automatically mean that you will learn something as a result of the experience. You must actually want to learn something. This means that the difference between an experience and a learning experience is you. Learning will not happen by osmosis; it starts and ends with you.

If you have the drive, determination and motivation to learn through all the practice experiences you encounter, they will become learning experiences. However, if you fail to treat all your experiences as learning opportunities, your practice experience will mean little to you and countless learning opportunities will be lost. This would be the equivalent of sleepwalking through practice (Elcock, 2006) – your body may have been there, but your brain has been asleep.

Activity 5.3 — *Reflection*

In Activity 5.1 you were required to indentify predictable and unpredictable learning experiences at the initial interview. As you progress through your practice experience you should endeavour to identify new opportunities for learning that you may become aware of. The midpoint interview provides a great opportunity not only to reconsider your learning needs with your mentor, but also to discuss new and additional learning experiences. As these opportunities occur to you, it's useful to document these in either your practice assessment document or practice portfolio. Use the grid to make a note of new learning experiences that may occur during a practice experience.

Predictable Experiences	Unpredictable Experiences

continued opposite . . .

continued . . .

Predictable Experiences	Unpredictable Experiences

As this activity is for your own reflection, there is no outline answer at the end of the chapter.

A plan for learning

No learning will happen unless you are clear about what it is you would like to learn. The learning outcomes that you bring to your practice experience will already supply you with this information. Remember that these learning objectives are derived from the *Standards for Pre-registration Nursing Education* (NMC, 2010). This means that what you need to learn is based on what the NMC requires you to learn, so this needs to be taken very seriously. Understanding what you are required to learn should form part of the preparation for your practice experience and the whole of Chapter 3 was dedicated to this theme. If you really want to learn in practice, thorough preparation before you arrive is essential.

Case study

Ann has been allocated a practice experience in an oncology day-care clinic. To prepare for this experience, Ann reads through the ten learning outcomes in her practice assessment document. One of her learning outcomes reads as follows:

Learning Outcome 7

Demonstrate sensitivity to the diverse care needs of patients and clients when planning and managing care.

In the weeks leading up to her practice experience, Ann puts some time into her preparation. Her university has a practice education website, and she makes a point of working through the online pre-practice activities and also visits the clinic to introduce herself to her mentor. She realises that she will be caring for a wide age range of patients and looks forward to this challenge. Ann arrives for her first day of practice ready to learn.

Experiential learning

By the time you arrive for your practice experience you should have already planned, and be clear about, what you want to learn, as in the case study. However, you also need to plan how you are going to learn. Without a clear plan of how to do this, learning experiences will be lost. You will need to plan how you will learn through your experiences by using a process in which there is an active and interactive process between the learner and the environment (Dewey, 1933). This process is broadly referred to as **experiential learning**.

There are many experiential learning cycles and theories that you may have already heard about in terms of nursing education. It is simply not possible to look at each of these different theories within this book, nor is it necessary. The main point is that a learning cycle provides a purposeful and realistic way to learn in, through and during the experiences you will encounter in practice. As an added bonus, it is quite simple to learn how to accept responsibility for your learning experiences by using a learning cycle.

Kolb's experiential learning cycle

Kolb's (1984) process of experiential learning is an easy way for you to start planning how to learn in, through and during an experience. His model of experiential learning is best described as a four-stage cycle of different learning modes. Figure 5.1 shows each stage of the cycle clearly. A great feature of the experiential cycle is that each stage – concrete experience, reflective observation, abstract conceptualisation and active experimentation (Kolb, 1984) – represents a different aspect of what you might learn during a learning experience.

Concrete experience

You may find that your learning experiences often begin at the concrete experience stage of the learning cycle. This essentially happens because a concrete experience is where you have the opportunity to do something (Dennison and Kirk, 1990). The great part about practice is that you don't have to conjure up your concrete experiences; they occur constantly and you will have no trouble in finding them. Have a look back at Activity 5.1 on page 66. Every single predictable and unpredictable experience that you listed could be classed as a concrete experience.

You will only learn during a concrete experience if you make links between the experience itself and your learning outcomes (Cantor, 1995). If you have prepared for practice thoroughly, you should have a very clear understanding of the types of concrete experiences you will need to have during your practice experience in order to meet learning outcomes. When these events do arise, you will be able to identify them straight away and latch on to them as learning opportunities.

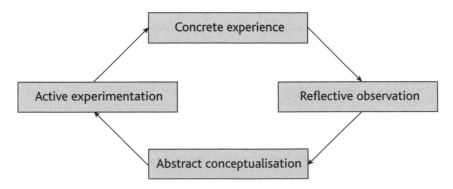

Figure 5.1: Kolb's experiential learning cycle (adapted from Kolb, 1984, p42)

Activity 5.4 — *Reflection*

Think back to a recent concrete learning experience you have had during a practice learning opportunity. Use the space below to describe the event, but also what you felt you were learning during the event. In particular, try to consider any conscious reflection you did during the concrete experience. If you are aware of any reflection that you took place during the event, what difference do you think this made to your learning experience?

As this activity is for your own reflection, there is no outline answer at the end of the chapter.

You may have realised, when completing Activity 5.4, that you did not consciously reflect during the event. If this is the case, this may have limited your learning experience. In order to learn during a concrete experience you will also need to reflect on the experience while the experience is happening. In the theory element of your course you will already have been introduced to reflection as a process of deep thought that includes looking backwards to the situation being pondered upon and projecting forward to the future (Carroll et al., 2001).

Jarvis (1992) argues that reflective practice is more than just thoughtful practice; it is the process of turning thoughtful practice into a potential learning situation. Schön (1983) calls this 'reflection-in-action'. It is ideally suited to being utilised within a concrete experience as it involves looking at past experiences, individual values, opinions and expectations in order to handle a current situation; in other words, it is 'thinking on your feet' (Pattison et al., 2000). If you fail to reflect during a concrete learning experience, it will be very difficult to move on to the next stage of the learning cycle, and the value of the experience will be lost.

Case study

Ann's practice experience gets off to a great start and she is enjoying all the different learning opportunities available. During her first week she identifies activities that will provide her with opportunities to meet her learning outcomes. Every Wednesday the morning clinic is set aside for adolescents who are undergoing chemotherapy. She decides to use the activities that take place during this clinic to focus on Learning Outcome 7 (see the previous case study on page 69), as a range of therapeutic approaches is used to care for the patients. During one of these clinics Ann has the opportunity to care for Carlos, a 14-year-old boy who is nearing the

continued overleaf . . .

continued . . . .

end of his treatment programme. Carlos is experiencing ongoing nausea as a result of his chemotherapy and is distressed about losing his hair.

Ann listens as her mentor, Fiona, gives him advice about anti-emetics, explaining how the medications work and the best time to take them. Fiona takes her time with Carlos, giving him the opportunity to express his feelings rather than rushing off to the next patient. When Carlos discloses that his main concern is losing his hair, Fiona talks to him about a support group for teenagers that he could attend. Ann realises that Fiona is gradually building a rapport with Carlos, and that her communication skills are essential to the care she is providing. Ann asks if she can talk to Fiona about Carlos, and they decide to talk in the afternoon as the morning clinic is very busy.

Reflective observation

The next stage in Kolb's experiential learning cycle is a more formalised type of reflection that occurs after the concrete experience event. If a concrete experience can be defined as 'doing', the reflective observation stage is more attune to 'reviewing' (Dennison and Kirk, 1990). In this stage there is a need to reflect on and observe the experiences you have had from many perspectives (Kolb, 1984). In other words, learning occurs through a 'reflection-on-action'. According to Schön (1983), the reflection-on-action that takes place after a concrete experience must be guided so that thinking and practice can be moved forward. Ghaye and Lillyman (2000) contribute to this discussion by suggesting that a reflective conversation should occur following a 'reflection-in-action' event. While this may be perfectly reasonable in theory, the reality of practice means that you may find it very difficult to schedule a reflective conversation with your mentor after every concrete learning experience.

Case study

On Wednesday afternoon, Ann and Fiona take their tea break together and talk about the events of the morning. Ann is keen to talk about Carlos and they spend some time reviewing his history, and how his current treatment is resulting in unpleasant side effects. Ann describes how she felt when Carlos disclosed his concerns, and Fiona explains how she had decided to spend more time with Carlos as she could sense he was feeling very anxious. Fiona also discusses the need to communicate sensitively with teenagers, who are understandably affected by changes to their body image. They debate the different techniques used in the clinic for treating nausea and hair loss, and Ann is fascinated to learn that massage is used by some patients to reduce their anxiety. At the end of the tea break Ann realises that there is far more she would like to learn on the subject.

While formal reflection may be difficult due to the busyness of practice areas, in most situations it will be possible to undertake informal reflection following practice events with your mentor. Ghaye and Lillyman (2008) suggest that this can be achieved by 'reflection-through-practice' and through reflection for the improvement of practice. You will need to assume responsibility for these reflective sessions, either by prompting your mentor to discuss the experience straight away or negotiating a convenient time to reflect together. Either way, this will take some motivation on your part, especially as the ability to reflect is the skill in which many adult learners are deficient (Duley, 1980). The main point is that you do undertake some form of reflection on your practice, as Ghaye et al. (1996) believe that, without reflection, it is often impossible to improve practice. Therefore, it can also be argued that, without reflection, it is impossible to learn. In fact, Pattison et al. (2000) go as far as to say that, if we do not embrace reflection, we will never have the opportunity to question the values that underpin our practice and make us the healthcare professionals we claim to be.

Reflecting during the practice experience

There are many different ways in which you could use reflection during your practice experience. Take some time now to read through the different types of reflection that may be available to you.

- **Descriptive reflection** The individual's personal, comprehensive, retrospective account of a situation.
- **Perceptive reflection** Contains explanations for the feelings of the individual.
- **Receptive reflection** Reflection-on-action. Provides a justification for practice and offers a link between the individual's thinking, feelings and practice, and those of others.
- **Interactive reflection** Reflection shows a link between learning from reflection and future action. A rationale for action is given with the aim of moving practice forward.
- **Critical reflection** Reflection-on-practice. Challenges the status quo and examines the structures that serve to liberate or constrain practice.

Source: Adapted from Pattison et al. (2000, p76)

Abstract conceptualisation

The abstract conceptualisation stage of the experiential learning cycle relates to the thought processes that take place and the subsequent knowledge that you will attain following the concrete experience and your reflective observation. There is no real, set formula to what and how you should 'abstractedly conceptualise', as it is your opportunity to make sense of the learning experience following your reflection. It is a bit like a re-evaluation of the experience, in which Boud and Walker (1993) suggest that you can link current experiences with past experiences, integrate the current experience into what you currently know, test for validity and then turn it into your own learning.

It is at this stage of the learning cycle that you may be able to identify your specific strengths and weaknesses, or gaps in your knowledge that need to be addressed. In fact, reflective observation and abstract conceptualisation tend to merge naturally into each other, as it is almost impossible to pinpoint when reflection becomes new insight and vice versa. Pattison et al. (2000) suggest that it is this continuum of reflective practices that distinguishes a nurse from a technician. Yet the main point is that learning takes place as a result of abstract conceptualisation, because you are able to create concepts that integrate your observations into logically sound theories (Kolb, 1984). It is this movement through the learning cycle that allows for learning in, through and during experiences.

Case study

After talking with Fiona, Ann realises that she would like to learn more about the support and advice available for adolescents with cancer. Over the course of the next week, she makes a point of attending a multidisciplinary team (MDT) meeting and has the opportunity to observe a teenage support group meeting where relaxation techniques, including aromatherapy and massage, are available. She also realises that her knowledge of chemotherapy and anti-emetic medications is limited and she uses some practice time to study the literature and increase her knowledge of the medications.

Active experimentation

The last stage of Kolb's experiential learning cycle is defined as active experimentation and, as the term suggests, this part of the cycle is event orientated. In fact, on the surface it is very similar to the concrete experience stage as it involves an activity or event. However, active experimentation is not just concerned with the event or experience itself. It is the application stage of the cycle where the emphasis is on practical applications as opposed to reflective understanding; there is a pragmatic concern with what works, on influencing people and changing situations (Kolb, 1984). In other words, active experimentation is all about applying knowledge. You experience an event, you think about it, you make sense of what happened and then you adjust your practices as a result of what you have learned. Dennison and Kirk (1990) propose that, if the learning cycle up to this point has been successful, you will have the capacity and understanding to act differently.

It is important to note that, while active experimentation is the last stage of the learning cycle, it provides the opportunity for a new beginning rather than an end. By moving through a complete learning cycle you will be capable of behaving in a way that you would not have known previously when you are next confronted with a new situation (Dennison and Kirk, 1990). Your experiences of moving through one cycle will naturally open up opportunities to engage with new concrete experiences that will start another cycle all over again. Perhaps this is best summed up by Kolb (1984) in his assertion that we can all learn from our experiences and the results of this learning will pull us through.

Case study

The following Wednesday, Carlos returns to the day-care clinic. Ann works with Fiona to set up his chemotherapy and is pleased to find that she now has a better understanding of why the chemotherapy must be

continued opposite . . .

---

continued . . . ▸ ●●

given in a certain order. Carlos mentions that his nausea has been reduced and his appetite has improved. Ann talks to him about his new chemotherapy regime and, as his treatment progresses through the morning, she is able to answer most of his questions. Ann's experience with Carlos has made her recognise the importance of establishing trust, being sensitive to the needs of her patients and, most importantly, treating each patient as an individual. Now that she has learned some of these skills, she decides to get more involved in support groups for patients in the day-care clinic. She discusses her options with Fiona and arranges to shadow one of the nurse specialists the next day.

Planning experiential learning

It is very important to understand that planning of learning experiences does not just take place at the beginning of each practice event. Of course, thorough planning at the initial interview is very important, as is the midpoint review, but your learning will be very limited if you do not continue to review all experiences through the entire practice learning opportunity. The experiential learning cycle provides an opportunity to reflect on different learning needs and available opportunities. As you complete each cycle of learning you should aim to uncover additional learning experiences available to you and make additional plans for how to learn through these experiences. In the next chapter we will look at documenting your learning experience as evidence that learning has taken place.

Your style of learning

Not only does Kolb's experiential learning cycle (Kolb, 1984) provide a comprehensive plan for learning, it also allows you to blend your preferred learning style into the learning cycle. You should already have a clear understanding of your preferred learning style, and also the style of learning that is least like you. We dealt with this in Chapter 2. Remember that you will need to use facets of all learning styles in order to make the most of your learning opportunities and also develop competence. Kolb's learning cycle makes this possible, as each stage of the learning cycle matches one type of learning style. In Figure 5.2, it should be clear that each part of the learning cycle supports a different type of learning style.

This means that every learning activity that you engage with in practice will have at least one aspect that matches your own preferred learning style. Therefore, if you are a theorist you may choose to begin your learning cycle at the abstract conceptualisation stage; likewise, an activist may choose to begin their learning at the concrete experience stage. It is important to remember that there is no right or wrong way to begin a learning cycle; the most important thing is that you do move sequentially through each stage of the cycle to ensure that you have made the most of each opportunity. This will give you a chance to practise and develop the learning style that you least prefer and, in so doing, move towards developing your nursing competence.

Figure 5.2: Kolb's experiential learning cycle and learning style (adapted from Kolb, 1984, p42, and Honey and Mumford, 1992, p7)

Chapter summary

We all have the potential to learn in, through and during experiences. However, learning doesn't just happen by itself. In order to learn from your practice experiences, you will first need to want to learn, and then deliberately set out to learn. Kolb's experiential learning cycle provides an opportunity to completely engage with a learning experience during all stages of your practice learning experience. Not only will learning become more enjoyable, but your experiences and subsequent reflections will open up a world of future learning opportunities that will stimulate further learning. The rewards will be immediate, and the effort you put into your learning will be paid back to you – with interest.

Further reading

Dennison, B and Kirk, R (1990) *Do, Review, Learn, Apply: A simple guide to experiential learning.* Oxford: Blackwell Education.

This book provides an easy-to-read overview of experiential learning, with simple descriptions of theory and practical examples and case studies.

Useful websites

www.learningandteaching.info/learning/experience.htm

This website provides a great overview of the experiential learning model and its relationship to learning styles.

www.businessballs.com/kolblearningstyles.htm

A detailed look at Kolb's experiential learning cycle with suggestions on how to incorporate learning styles into a learning sequence.

Chapter 6
Independent learning in practice

continued overleaf . . .

continued . . . .

individual situation promoting health and well-being, minimising risk of harm and promoting their safety at all times.

14. People can trust the newly registered graduate nurse to be autonomous and confident as a member of the multi-disciplinary or multi-agency team and to inspire confidence in others.

15. People can trust the newly registered graduate nurse to safely delegate to others and to respond appropriately when a task is delegated to them.

Chapter aims

The aim of this chapter is to provide an insight into the benefit and process of independent learning in practice.

After reading this chapter you will be able to:

- understand the main principles of self-regulated learning and the specific challenges of learning in practice;
- appreciate the importance of interviews, feedback and documentation in relation to competence;
- recognise the role of your mentor in their contribution to your learning experience.

Introduction: independent learning – setting the scene

In the previous chapter, we discussed the need to plan your learning experiences throughout your practice in order to gain maximum benefit. We now know that learning experiences should be planned before the initial interview and reviewed consistently throughout your practice period. There will be an opportunity to review your learning opportunities formally at the midpoint interview with your mentor; however, you should not rely just on this one event. This is especially true if your learning experience involves rotating through a number of practice areas, as experiences will constantly be changing.

We now know that the motivation to prepare for a practice experience is largely dependent on your ability to learn as an adult, but it also involves the skill of self-regulated learning. The ability to be a self-regulated learner is important not only for practice preparation; it is also a vital skill to master in order to create the best possible learning opportunities during your practice experiences. Without this skill you could find yourself struggling to cope with the practice elements of your course, as these will have been designed for an adult learner.

The focus of this chapter will be on exploring the nature of self-regulation skills in relation to practice, and ways in which these skills can be developed to your advantage. The starting point is to define 'self-regulation' and how this is applicable to the practice learning environment. There will be an opportunity to investigate the particular challenges of practice learning, and how to be a self-regulated learner to meet these challenges. We will then consider the importance of the assessment process, feedback and documentation in relation to competence. Finally, there will be an opportunity to explore the role of your mentor in terms of their contribution to your independent learning experience.

Self-regulated learning

Self-regulation is fundamentally a state of being, rather than a state of doing. While self-direction involves the function of organising your learning, self-regulated learning is focused on using your own motivation and drive to develop your own learning experience. Sung (2006) explains that self-regulated learners set their own task-specific learning goals and employ appropriate strategies to attain these goals. These may be very different from the self-directed activities you may have already engaged in, where the learning goal may have been given to you. These may include self-study days or activities such as problem-based learning, blended learning, practice learning logs or independent learning contracts (Smedley, 2007). In fact, study for exams or assignment preparation may also be classed as a self-directed activity.

In this context, 'self-direction' is a euphemism for undertaking a task or activity with minimum supervision. While such a skill is commendable, it is important to recognise that there is a clear distinction between *doing* a self-directed activity, and *being* a self-regulated learner. While the difference may appear subtle, in reality they are worlds apart. It is important to recognise that gaining the most from your practice learning opportunities will require you to develop and master the skills of self-regulated learning. In essence, this means that you will need to demonstrate the skills of independent learning in practice.

Learning in theory, learning in practice

It is not uncommon for students to put a great deal of effort into addressing academic challenges, assuming that the skills they attain while undertaking the theory programme will readily transfer to the practice environment. However, the challenges of the practice environment are very different from the types of issues you may encounter during your theory work. These different challenges mean that you will need to develop a new range of skills to learn during practice. You will essentially be required to demonstrate competence in a wide range of areas, such as knowledge development, critical understanding, practical skills, and professional values and standards (Flanagan et al., 2000). In Chapter 4 (Figure 4.1, page 57) we identified that learning in practice requires the ability to apply, under supervision, a combination of cognitive, psychomotor and affective skills to solve problems and make clinical decisions (Windsor, 1987). In Figure 4.1, these three aspects of competence were termed 'knowledge', 'skills' and 'attitude'.

So the skills that you will need for learning in practice will be vastly different from the skills you may have developed during theoretical coursework.

Activity 6.1	*Communication*

We already know that learning in theory is different from learning in practice. If you have already undertaken a practice experience, you will be familiar with some of the differences. Use this table to note down the different challenges you have already faced or think you may face in practice as opposed to the theoretical part of your course. Try to think specifically about the skills you may need for each environment and how these may differ. An example has been provided to get you started.

Current skills in theory learning	**Challenges of practice learning**
Presenting information during a tutorial session to classmates I know well.	Presenting information during a team meeting to practice staff I don't know at all.

This activity will provide you with the opportunity to identify the areas of practice experience that may require additional preparation, for example accessing additional practice resources or setting yourself individual learning goals.

An outline of the differences is given at the end of the chapter.

Take some time to reflect on the list you have compiled in Activity 6.1, as some of the challenges for practice learning may be quite surprising. Just because you are confident in one skill in theory does not mean you will be able to transfer the same confidence to practice. The good news is that, once you understand your learning needs, you can learn how to transfer your skills to cope with these challenges.

Learning skills

We spend our whole lives learning new skills and putting these skills into practice in a variety of situations. In fact, we have learned so many skills during the course of our lifetimes that we take many of them for granted. We use some skills so often during the course of a normal day that we don't even think consciously about the skill at all while we are using it. For example, you are reading this book, and reading is a pretty amazing skill. You had to be taught how to read, and at first this was probably quite difficult as you learned all the different letters and sounds. However, now that you have learned to read, it is unlikely that you think about the process at all, as it just becomes an automatic part of your life.

Activity 6.2	*Reflection*

Stop for a minute and think about all the times today when you used your reading skills, then use the box below to make a list.

The ways I have used my reading skills today include . . .

As this activity is for your own reflection, there is no outline answer at the end of the chapter.

You may have had to think hard about the list you compiled in Activity 6.2, and no doubt you have probably forgotten to include quite a few obvious situations. For example, did you remember to include reading the shopping list on your fridge door, or the name of the TV programme you set to record on your Sky box? What about the street signs on your satnav, or the message from your friend on Facebook? The truth is that you are able to use your reading skills all day every day without consciously thinking about them. You have learned how to transfer your reading skills into a wide range of different situations.

Low-road transfer

When skills that you have developed become automatic and part of your subconscious, this is referred to as **low-road transfer** (Salomon and Perkins, 1989). Using low-road transfer you are able to apply your skills with very little in the way of mindfulness or conscious deliberation (Sung, 2006). In other words, you are able to do something without having to think about it. Have a look again at the list you created in Activity 6.2 regarding the times you used your reading skills today. Now imagine if you had to think about how to read before actually reading something. No doubt you would be quite frustrated, and may have missed out on some important events. The point is that the ability to employ low-road transfer actually helps in adapting and functioning quickly within a variety of situations without getting bogged down in detail or needing to analyse each separate event. The main benefit of low-road transfer is that the more varied the situations in which you utilise a certain skill, the more automatic the application becomes (Sung, 2006).

Scenario

Driving a car is frequently used as an example of low-road transfer. When you first learn to drive you are very conscious of every action, and also very aware of other traffic on the road. You have to think through all actions you take to ensure you coordinate them in the correct order. As time progresses and you develop driving experience you start to become more automatic in your actions. Eventually, you find yourself driving a car without actually being aware of your actions. In fact, you can arrive at a destination without being conscious of what you did to get there, as the whole experience has become a low-road transfer skill.

High-road transfer

Of course, the opposite of low-road transfer is **high-road transfer**. Salomon and Perkins (1989) describe high-road transfer as a way of examining a situation, then deciding on an alternative action when faced with an unfamiliar task. For example, while you might use low-road transfer to read a book, you will need high-road transfer to understand and make sense of what you are reading. The fact is that you will have to employ high-road transfer skills in order to become a self-regulated learner in practice. While low-road transfer skills are primarily focused on getting the job done, high-road transfer skills allow you to question why you are doing the job. In order to be independent in your practice learning, you must strive to develop and maintain a high-road transfer approach within your learning experience. While low-road transfer may help you to perform a task adequately, high-road transfer will prompt you to question why you are performing the task. In other words, while low-road transfer is about doing, high-road transfer is about knowing why you do.

Case study

Dev is undertaking his practice experience in a medical ward. One of his outcomes for the practice experience was to demonstrate competence in administering subcutaneous injections. Every day he has had the opportunity to undertake this skill and his mentor has indicated that he is competent with his injection technique. Dev has become so confident that he does not really think about the task any more, as it has become routine.

One morning, Dev is being supervised by his mentor on the medication round and begins to prepare a subcutaneous injection for his patient. His mentor stops him and enquires about the patient's blood sugar recording. Dev has not thought to look at the chart; he has been so focused on performing the task that he has not checked to see if the medication should be given. The patient's chart is checked and it becomes clear that the injection is no longer required. If Dev had proceeded with the injection, this would have resulted in patient harm

continued opposite . . .

continued . . .

and a serious medication error. It becomes clear to Dev and his mentor that, while he may have learned to perform an injection competently, he does not have the knowledge of managing the safe care of his patient.

Dev has made the classic mistake of confusing 'doing a skill' with competence. He has forgotten that competence is an equal mix of skill, knowledge and attitude. By focusing only on the ability to undertake the skill, Dev has demonstrated low-road transfer, but by not knowing why he is undertaking the skill, or considering his patient's welfare, he is not demonstrating high-road transfer. Dev is not competent as he has not demonstrated evidence of skills, knowledge and attitude.

High-road transfer and self-regulation

From the above, we can see that there is a very strong link between high-road transfer and self-regulation. If you adopt low-road transfer during your practice experiences, your learning experience will become a sequence of tasks and activities that you move from and to with little understanding of why you are performing the tasks, or the significance of those tasks. Even worse, your learning will be dictated by the availability of tasks, and when these specific activities are not supplied you may find yourself at a loss and feeling as if you do not know what to do. This is because you see your role as a doer, rather than a knowledgeable doer. So high-road transfer is vital because it allows you to comprehend the appropriateness of applying a previously acquired skill in an entirely new situation (Sung, 2006). It will be your ability to utilise high-road transfer that will provide opportunities for demonstrating your competence within the unpredictability of the practice environment. Sung (2006) argues that your ability to use conscious deliberation with only limited guidance is more likely to produce real understanding, rather than the formulaic learning that results from repetition and extended practice.

Self-regulation and the NMC

The NMC makes it very clear that the requirement for nurses to be self-regulated in their practice is not negotiable. Among other requirements, in order to achieve fitness for practice, a registered nurse must demonstrate the ability to search the evidence base, disseminate research findings and adapt practice where necessary (NMC, 2010). These requirements are entirely self-regulatory and are implicit within the domain of professional accountability and responsibility. As a consequence, Zimmerman (1995) highlights that self-regulated learning encapsulates three distinct phases: planning, performance and evaluation. It is no coincidence that such skills are synonymous with the need to reflect on practice that is required for safe and competent care within a work-based learning context (Flanagan et al., 2000). These are also the skills related to high-road transfer. Reflection on practice does not fit with a low-road transfer approach. You will need to be self-regulated in order to demonstrate your competence for qualification.

Learning independently

In the last chapter we established that Kolb's experiential learning cycle provides ongoing opportunities to plan and undertake learning experiences in practice (Kolb, 1984). We also established that the opportunities for learning will need to be constantly reviewed throughout a practice experience to ensure that learning experiences are being optimised.

The point of being a self-regulated learner is that it will be your responsibility to engage in, review and record your learning experiences. Just as you take responsibility to review your learning opportunities throughout your practice experience, you will need to alter, change or revise your learning experiences as you encounter new opportunities.

The initial interview is your opportunity to discuss with your mentor the types of learning experiences you would like to have. Of course, this discussion will largely be based on your understanding of the experiences that are available. In Chapter 5 we looked at some activities that demonstrated a way to identify learning opportunities throughout the practice experience. If you have prepared thoroughly for the practice experience, you should have a very clear understanding of what you need to achieve during the practice experience and some examples of activities that you would like to take part in. Likewise, as your practice period continues you will become aware of new opportunities that can be added into your learning plan and used to undertake learning cycles. The midpoint interview is a key time to review your learning experiences, so you should take full advantage of this time with your mentor to review, change and develop your learning experiences.

Case study

Jacqui reflects on learning independently in practice.

In the first week I was able to meet with my mentor and she asked me what I wanted to do while I was in their GUM clinic. I think she got a bit of a shock when I opened my assessment document and showed her that I had written a brief plan next to all the learning outcomes. I'd already researched the clinic by looking at their profile on the practice website, so I'd gone ahead and selected the outcomes I wanted to achieve and also what experiences I wanted to do in order to achieve the outcomes. For example, there was an outcome about written communication and I put in my plan that I wanted to write up care plans and document in the clients' files. My mentor was really impressed, especially when I explained that I'd appreciate it if we could reflect on my documentation and she could give me feedback on what areas I needed to develop. I also explained that I wanted to have lots of different communication experiences, so I could demonstrate competence in all the written records they kept. At the end of my third week I realised that the clinic maintained online records, so I discussed this with my mentor and we set a new plan for how I could be involved in this. At the midpoint, we reviewed this plan again and set new goals of me being able to access blood results

continued opposite . . .

continued . . .

and also fill out the forms for SDI screening. I learned so much and had the best experience, mainly because I took responsibility right from the start. My mentor was really encouraging and supported all the learning experiences I wanted to involve myself with, but, ultimately, it was down to me to work out what I wanted to do and take control of my own learning.

Evidence of learning

As you move through each practice experience your learning experiences will need to be recorded. There may be an opportunity to record your experiences in your practice assessment document or practice portfolio. It will be your responsibility to maintain these records and ensure they accurately reflect your experiences. Very often, what you document will be used by your mentor to discuss your progress during the practice experience and even as a basis for practice assessment. A clear record of your learning experiences can ensure that your midpoint interview becomes a focused discussion on your achievements so far, as well as your ongoing learning needs for the remainder of the practice experience. Keeping documented records of your practice experiences ensures that you have a clear record of your progress and can plan future learning experiences. As an independent learner, it will be your responsibility to maintain these records and ensure that they are detailed enough to be of value. If you are not being exposed to the learning experiences you need, a detailed practice portfolio will provide evidence of what deficits there have been. This is especially important if you move through a variety of practice areas. The more detailed your portfolio, the more information your primary mentor will have regarding your progress at the times they are indirectly observing you during the practice experience.

An example of an entry within a practice learning portfolio is provided in Figure 6.1.

A portfolio is also a great way to assess your own developmental progress and focus your efforts on your ongoing learning needs. If a practice experience lasts over many weeks, it will be impossible for you to remember every learning experience you have been involved with; neither

Monday, 23rd May 2011 – Today I cared for two children with measles. I had experience with medicine administration, assessment and observations. There was also an opportunity to develop my competence in infection control and fluid management. I found it difficult to communicate with one mother as she was very anxious and questioned everything I did. I'd like to develop my skills in communicating with parents, especially when they are confrontational.

Tuesday, 24th May 2011 – Today I worked alongside a school nurse. We were able to discuss signs and symptoms of measles, and also how immunisation records are kept in the UK. I'd like to find out more about educating parents about immunisation, and also possible complications such as pneumonia.

Figure 6.1: Practice learning portfolio

will you remember your reaction or role in that learning event. A portfolio can therefore be used as a basis for later reflection, and even be incorporated into a professional development portfolio.

When do I document?

You will probably be provided with instructions from your university on the frequency of maintaining records in your portfolio. For example, this may be daily or weekly. Try to maintain your records as soon as possible after the learning event so that it remains fresh and you can recall any immediate feelings or feedback you have received. Not only will you be demonstrating an independent approach to your learning (Sung, 2006), you will also be able to identify quickly if learning experiences are not meeting your learning needs and take measures to rectify this. In addition, documentation of your own records will be helping you develop written communication skills, an NMC requirement for competence (NMC, 2010). If your portfolio is in a folder or booklet, get into the habit of taking this to practice with you. If your portfolio is online, ask your mentor if you can have access to the local computer to update your portfolio at the end of the shift. To be of value, the portfolio needs to record evidence of your learning experiences and be available for review by you and your mentor throughout the practice experience.

Self-regulation and your mentor

Many students return from their practice experiences disappointed and feeling as if they have learned nothing (Elcock, 2006). It is not uncommon for students to feel as if they are being used as 'just a pair of hands', blaming their mentors for limited learning experiences. As we have discussed already in this chapter, as you should be an independent learner your mentor does not have sole responsibility or accountability for your learning. This is a shared experience, so you should be prepared to regulate your own learning experiences.

The fact is that some students do not take advantage of all potential learning experiences as they are waiting to be told what to do, either by their mentor or through information provided by the university. However, your mentor is only required to *provide* a learning experience and opportunity for you. If you do not take advantage of the experiences and opportunities available to you, this is not your mentor's fault. In terms of your learning experiences, as long as your mentor is fulfilling their role in relation to the *Standards for Learning and Assessment in Practice* (NMC, 2008b), the rest is up to you.

Case study

A mentor speaks about the pleasure of working with students who demonstrate self-regulation skills.

You can always tell the really keen students. They're the ones that are always asking questions and don't hang around waiting to be told what to do. They get stuck in, and you find that you want to spend more time explaining things because they obviously

continued opposite . . .

continued . . .

want to learn and put the effort in themselves. They know what they want to learn, and don't expect me to do the learning for them. I'll go out of my way for these students, because you know they are really trying hard and want to learn as much as possible.

If a student comes to the initial interview with a list of experiences they want, then I know what I've got to do. I can arrange for them to attend a home visit with the discharge team for example, if that's what they want to do. If they come to me at the midpoint and say they would like to spend a day with the ITU outreach nurse, then I'll sort that out as well. I can't know what they need unless they tell me. I'm not a mind reader, so if a student doesn't let me know what they need, how am I supposed to know?

The practice environment is packed with potential learning opportunities, so virtually every activity that takes place has the potential to be turned into a learning experience. Kelly et al. (2007) recommend that you are up-front with your mentor about what you want to learn during your practice experience, and what you are already competent in doing. It is your awareness and insight into your own learning needs that will form the basis of self-regulation. Therefore, if you show a genuine interest and enthusiasm from the start, this will pay dividends throughout the practice experience. Remember, though, that you will only be able to speak knowledgeably about your learning outcomes if you have prepared thoroughly for practice.

Activity 6.3   *Team working*

Take some time to speak with a selection of your colleagues regarding their experiences of learning in practice. If possible, try to sample students from a number of different stages of the pre-registration programme. Ask them to nominate ways that they have successfully been able to negotiate learning experiences with mentors. Make some notes in the space below. In particular, look for common themes or approaches that have worked in the past and led to successful learning experiences. What can you learn from your colleagues that could improve your own practice experience?

_____

_____

_____

_____

As this activity is based on your own observation, there is no outline answer at the end of the chapter.

In undertaking Activity 6.3 you will also have been developing your ability to work with a team of people towards a common goal. As the NMC requires that you must *work effectively across professional and agency boundaries, respecting and making the most of contributions made by others to achieve integrated person centred care* (NMC, 2010), this is an ideal way to practise that skill with your colleagues. The activity will also have helped you to develop your communication skills, as we discussed earlier in the chapter. You could have considered doing this activity within a class discussion or setting up an online discussion in a message board. The experiences you share could benefit not only yourself but everyone in the group who participates in the discussion.

Case study

Victoria and Mel are undertaking their practice experience in a care home. Victoria is having a very unhappy time as she feels she is learning nothing. Every day her mentor allocates her a small group of residents to care for and, although she has been practising skills of personal care and communication, she feels let down that there is not more to learn. She spends a lot of time sitting in the day room looking through patient notes and wishing she was in a more dynamic learning environment. She has asked to leave early several times when she feels that there is nothing for her to learn.

Mel is learning far more than she could have expected. As well as caring for her residents, she makes time every day to participate in the medication round with her mentor, and has been able to learn about the actions of at least three major drug groupings. She has asked to spend a day shadowing the physiotherapist, and has been able to participate in team meetings and lead a therapy group. Every day she sets herself new goals of what she would like to learn and discusses with her mentor how best to meet her goals.

At the midpoint review, Mel shares her portfolio with her mentor and asks if they can plan some new learning experiences, including accompanying residents to outpatient clinics at the local hospital and attending the senior managers' meeting. Mel's mentor quickly agrees that this would be a valuable experience and agrees to make the necessary arrangements. Victoria is very unhappy with her midpoint interview. She has not maintained a practice portfolio and she feels she has had very few learning experiences to record. Victoria's mentor reviews her outcomes and tells her she will continue to allocate her some residents every day.

At the end of her practice experience Mel achieves all her learning goals. Victoria does not achieve all her learning outcomes and her mentor recommends an additional practice period to help her achieve her goals. Victoria leaves the practice experience feeling that Mel received favoured treatment. She blames her mentor for not achieving her outcomes.

Activity 6.4   *Critical thinking*

Take some time to reflect on the above case study. What would you consider to be the main reason why Victoria failed to achieve all her outcomes? Is her belief that Mel received favoured treatment justified? Write some brief notes that will help you to think critically about the event.

An outline answer can be found at the end of the chapter.

Can I learn independently?

Your own expectations and experiences on entering the nursing programme will no doubt have some impact on your ability to be a self-regulated learner in practice. Nurse educators also play an important role in assisting students to apply their knowledge in the practice area (Beck, 1993). It is well recognised that nursing programmes do not always place enough emphasis on skills for self-regulated learning in practice. Universities are now providing practice orientation programmes that focus on the importance of self-regulatory learning strategies for student nurses (Mullen, 2007; Sharples and Moseley, 2010).

It may be that your current nursing course puts specific emphasis on helping you to develop self-regulation skills for learning in practice. This may even be referred to as 'learning to learn'. If this is the case, you are in a very fortunate position and should make the most of these development opportunities.

However, your ability to self-regulate your learning may also be related to your assumptions about the teaching you expect will be provided during the programme and your role in relation to learning. For example, some nursing students expect that their course will be teacher-directed and tightly structured (MacLeod, 1995). Like many students in the past, you may have entered the nursing course expecting to receive lectures, be provided with course material, involve yourself in some classroom discussion and complete the required assessments and exams (Wilkinson et al., 1998). If these were your expectations, you may have found the transition from being a passive recipient to being an active participant in your own learning quite daunting (Wilkinson et al., 1998). If this is true for you in the theory element of the course, learning in practice will be far more daunting in terms of your self-regulation skills.

Skills for self-regulated learning

You cannot expect to turn into a self-regulated learner overnight. Remember, this is a skill that will take considerable time and effort to master. To become self-regulated during your practice learning experience will require you to consider the types of activities that will be available to you, and also the feasibility of you taking part in these activities. You should also take your preferred learning style into account as well, as this will make the learning experience far more enjoyable. This may sound like a very complicated way to undertake seemingly simple learning experiences, but remember that you are aiming towards high-road transfer skills in order to become a knowledgeable doer. The good news is that self-regulation of learning can be easily mastered and adopted in order to learn through your practice experiences.

> **Chapter summary**
>
> The need to develop the skills of high-road transfer cannot be denied in terms of learning in practice. If you want to become a competent practitioner, you must provide evidence of self-regulated learning ability and such skills cannot be obtained without the use of high-
>
> *continued overleaf ...*

continued . . .

road transfer. There is a clear need, therefore, to develop your skills to learn independently in practice. Once you have developed the skills that support high-road transfer, you will be able to self-regulate your practice learning opportunities. The development of self-regulatory learning skills is the basis for learning in, through and during your practice experiences.

Activities: Brief outline answers

Activity 6.1 Learning in theory and learning in practice (page 80)

Current skills in theory learning	Challenges of practice learning
Presenting information during a tutorial session to classmates I know well.	Presenting information during a team meeting to practice staff I don't know at all.
In this experience you have the advantage of knowing the people you are presenting to, and no doubt have built up some close relationships within the group, so your friends will be supportive of your presentation.	In this experience you will be presenting in front of people that you don't know very well; they are not your friends and they will be assessing what you say and the way you present your information.
In addition, it is likely that you will have had some time to research the topic you are speaking about, and perhaps even rehearsed the presentation. Even if you are feeling nervous, all these factors will give you a degree of confidence during the presentation.	In addition, you may have had limited time to think about what you will be presenting and it is unlikely there has been an opportunity for rehearsal. You may have had no time at all to prepare what you will be saying as you could be required to provide information to a group based on a question or new query.

Development of communication skills is not just for your benefit; it will be an essential part of your professional requirement as a nurse. The requirement for competent communication and interpersonal skills is addressed within the NMC's *The Code: Standards of conduct, performance and ethics for nurses and midwives*, where it is stated that you must:

> *work with others to protect and promote the health and wellbeing of those in your care, their families and carers, and the wider community.*
> (2008a, p2)

Obviously, competent communication with others will play a key role in fulfilling this requirement.

Activity 6.4 Self-regulated learning (page 88)

This activity required you to analyse critically the case study involving the different practice experiences of Mel and Victoria. While there is no doubt that Victoria and Mel had different experiences, your answer should have considered the reason why this happened. Mel took a self-regulated approach to her practice experience and demonstrated evidence of planning and taking responsibility for practice learning. Her mentor responded to this approach and matched her enthusiasm. In contrast, Victoria demonstrated no interest in independent learning, and her mentor responded to this lack of enthusiasm. The fact is that Mel did not receive favoured treatment; she simply encouraged her mentor to respond to her practice experience with enthusiasm.

Further reading

Brockett, R and Hiemstra, R (1991) *Self-direction in Adult Learning: Perspectives on research and practice.* London: Routledge.

This book provides useful insight into the theory and research that underpins self-direction in relation to adult learning. The book offers strategies for applying the principles of self-direction and self-regulation in practice.

Useful websites

www.health.heacademy.ac.uk

The Higher Education Academy has a subject centre dedicated to health sciences and practice. Links to the Practice Learning and Support special interest group provide valuable information on current research and practices within practice learning environments.

Chapter 7
Using feedback to learn

```
╭─────────────────────────────────────────────────────────────────────╮
```

NMC Standards for Pre-registration Nursing Education

This chapter will address the following competencies:

Domain 3: Nursing practice and decision-making

4. All nurses must ascertain and respond to the physical, social and psychological needs of people, groups and communities. They must then plan, deliver and evaluate safe, competent and person-centred care in partnership with them, paying attention to changing health needs during different life stages, including progressive illness and death, loss and bereavement.
10. All nurses must evaluate their care to improve clinical decision making, quality and outcomes, using a range of methods, amending the plan of care, where necessary, and communicating changes to others.

Domain 4: Leadership, management and team working

8. All nurses must work effectively across professional and agency boundaries, actively involving and respecting others' contributions to integrated person-centred care. They must know when and how to communicate with and refer to other professionals and agencies in order to respect the choices of service users and others, promoting shared decision making, to deliver positive outcomes and to coordinate smooth, effective transition within and between services and agencies.

NMC Essential Skills Clusters

This chapter will address the following ESCs:

Cluster: Care, compassion and communication

4. People can trust a newly qualified graduate nurse to engage with them and their family or carers within their cultural environments in an acceptant and anti-discriminatory manner free from harassment and exploitation.

Cluster: Organisational aspects of care

12. People can trust the newly registered graduate nurse to respond to their feedback and a wide range of other sources to learn, develop and improve services.

> ## Chapter aims
>
> The aim of this chapter is to assist you with understanding the role of feedback in relation to your learning experience and assessment of competence.
>
> After reading this chapter you will be able to:
>
> * identify the key aspects of verbal and written feedback;
> * understand the relevance of feedback in facilitating learning;
> * appreciate the role of your mentor in delivering feedback.

Introduction: feedback

It is quite common for students in practice to receive lots of feedback from their mentor. Understandably, you will want to be given regular updates about your performance. As you are likely to be preoccupied with receiving a good report (Cahill, 1996), feedback can provide reassurance on your progress and an opportunity to improve if there are any problems. Ideally, you will want timely, balanced and respectful feedback (Kelly, 2007). To a certain extent you are reliant on your mentor to give feedback on your practice performance, so that you can improve your level of competence (Glover, 2000).

In this chapter we will be discussing how feedback is a vital aspect of your learning experience. We will start by looking at some common problems with feedback and the relationship between feedback and assessment, and you will also gain an insight into your mentor's role regarding feedback. The chapter will then explore why feedback is so important in helping you become a self-regulated learner. There will be an opportunity to reflect on your previous experiences in receiving feedback, and also to review when you should get feedback and the different types you can expect to receive. We will also look at the importance of understanding your own reactions to feedback in order to be able to learn from it. In addition, we will discuss how formal and informal feedback can be incorporated into a learning cycle. The chapter will conclude by looking at issues related to the documentation of feedback.

Problems with feedback

In the past, students have reported numerous problems with the feedback they receive from mentors. It is often given too late, is destructive rather than constructive, is personal in nature and fails to concentrate on skill (Cahill, 1996). When feedback fails to concentrate on skill development and enhanced clinical performance, it is typical for a student's reaction to become negative (Clynes and Raftery, 2008). For this reason, Dohrenwend (2002) points out that feedback should be an evaluation of performance, not an evaluation of character. It is clear, therefore, that mentors have a responsibility to deliver accurate and fair feedback. However, before you are tempted to become too judgemental and critical of mentors, it is worth looking at feedback from their perspective.

Assessment and feedback

An essential part of your assessment during practice experience requires your mentor to provide you with feedback. Your assessment will be undertaken using an assessment tool, with your mentor being required to provide an accurate and objective assessment of your competence (Chambers, 1998; Watson et al., 2002). While assessment documents vary according to your university, they invariably contain the same fundamental elements. There will be a section for recording the formal stages of initial, midpoint and final interviews. In addition, there will be an opportunity for you to make records of your practice learning experiences (either in the document or in a portfolio) and a section where feedback from your mentor can be recorded. As there is no fixed requirement from the NMC on how these elements should be structured, the written feedback you receive could be in the form of free text, tick boxes, or perhaps action and development plans.

In a study conducted by Gray and Smith (2000), students identified the provision of feedback as an attribute of a 'good' mentor. Yet, despite ample evidence to suggest the value and necessity of feedback within the mentoring role, there is also evidence to suggest that some mentors may be either failing to deliver feedback, or failing in the delivery of feedback. This is quite obviously of some concern, given that the provision of effective feedback is viewed as an essential element within the assessment process (RCN, 2005).

Failing to give feedback

For many mentors, giving feedback to students is one of the biggest challenges and most difficult aspects of their role. Many mentors find that the delivery of feedback is inhibited by the pressures of practice supervision, inadequate staffing levels, heavy workloads and lack of continuity of support (Aston and Molassiotis, 2003). There is a multitude of reasons why mentors fail to deliver feedback, the most common being:

- time restraints;
- competing clinical pressures;
- sick leave;
- night duty;
- annual leave.

Of course, the irony is that the periods of intense practice activity tend to be the moments when you will require maximum support and feedback (Clynes and Raftery, 2008). If a mentor fails to give feedback, this is a problem, as providing time for reflection, feedback, monitoring and documenting of a student's progress is a key responsibility of a mentor (RCN, 2007).

Student reactions to feedback

What you may not realise is that it is not uncommon for highly skilled and experienced mentors to experience fear at the thought of giving a student feedback. In fact, it is well known that some mentors have been so reluctant to give feedback to students that they have avoided doing it at all. Clynes and Raftery (2008) highlight that, despite careful preparation, some mentors may choose to delay or avoid evaluation meetings with students for fear of a negative response or overreaction to criticism.

Case study

It is the third week of Mary's practice experience and she is being supervised by her mentor, Denis, on a drug round. Denis has noticed on previous occasions that Mary struggles with drug calculations, and frequently forgets the formulas she should be using. He has pointed this out to her and has even offered to help with practising calculations on quiet shifts. Once again, during the drug round Mary struggles with her calculations and Denis decides to provide some feedback once the drug round is over. He is concerned that, if Mary does not show significant improvement, she will not achieve a competent standard. Mary reacts very badly to the feedback she receives from Denis. She accuses him of picking on her, as he has not spoken to other students about their drug calculations. She tells Denis that he puts too much pressure on her, and if he were not there she is sure she would be able to perform calculations. She decides that Denis 'has it in for her' and requests a new mentor.

The truth of the matter is that some students may not always accept a mentor's feedback, even if it is accurate, as they have a very poor understanding of their own level of performance. In the above case study, Mary feels that her treatment is unfair because she has no understanding of her learning needs. This means that, as a student, you must be prepared to receive all feedback, and not just the feedback that you wish to hear. It is not easy for your mentor to provide feedback, and almost impossible if you react badly to it.

The feedback you receive from a mentor is fundamentally based on their opinion. As a result, your feedback will be largely determined by:

- *what your mentor sees;*
- *how significant your mentor thinks it is;*
- *how your mentor interprets what they have seen;*
- *whether what your mentor sees may contribute to your current or future actions.*

(Eraut, 2006, p111)

Learning from feedback

The ability to learn and make use of the feedback you receive during practice experiences is once again related to your self-regulatory skills. Not only are you responsible for your learning, but you also have a responsibility to respond appropriately to the feedback you are given regarding your performance. We all want to hear the best about ourselves and, if feedback does not do this, there is a natural tendency to feel that it is inaccurate. This is not to say that you must believe automatically everything you are told, as mentors do not always get it right. However, you will need the skills to take on board the feedback you are given and evaluate your own performance objectively. Being able to self-assess your own performance is an advanced skill, but it is not impossible to learn and will only serve to enhance your own learning.

Johari window

A Johari window exercise (see Activity 7.1) is a great way to understand that there is more to you than the way you perceive or understand things. Each of the four windows represents an aspect of you – your personality – that is relevant to the way you view the world and others view you. It is a way of accepting who you are.

Activity 7.1   *Communication*

This activity allows you complete your own Johari window exercise. You will need to select a person to undertake this activity with; it should be someone who knows you well and is able to provide accurate insights.

Window 1 – Agree an aspect of you that you are both aware of.
Window 2 – Ask your friend to reveal something about you that you are not aware of.
Window 3 – Reveal something to your friend that they do not know about you.
Window 4 – Agree on an aspect of you that remains unknown (perhaps how you would react to an event that has never been experienced).

1. Known by self/ Known by others	**2. Unknown by self/ Known by others**
3. Known by self/ Unknown by others	**4. Unknown by self/ Unknown by others**

Source: Adapted from Dennison and Kirk (1990, p29)

In undertaking this activity you will be developing not only your communication skills but also your experience of feedback. Window 2 will allow your friend to give you feedback about one aspect of you that you are unaware of. How will you react to this feedback, especially if you learn something about yourself that makes you feel disappointed? Remember that, for feedback to be useful, it cannot always be what you want to hear; very often it will be related to an issue that you need to improve.

An outline answer is provided at the end of the chapter.

You may wonder what relevance the Johari window has to feedback during your practice experience. The simple answer is that, when you understand the principles of a Johari window, it becomes clear that you are not always the best judge of yourself. Some things that take place in practice will be clear and straightforward, and both you and your mentor may agree on some of your strengths and weaknesses (window 1). However, there will be things that your mentor will pick up about your performance in practice that you are unaware of (window 2). There will be reasons why you respond to certain situations in practice that only you understand (window 3). Finally, you will be exposed to new situations in practice that require you to take part in, or react to, a fresh experience (window 4). In all these instances, your mentor will be able to provide feedback, so you may end up hearing and learning brand new information about yourself that you have never realised. If you are prepared for this, you will stand a great chance of learning and developing from this feedback.

Past experiences of feedback

It may be that you have already had experiences of receiving feedback from a mentor. Some of those experiences may have been positive, and some may have been unsatisfactory. It is worth reflecting on previous experiences you may have had in receiving feedback, as this may highlight any issues you have in relation to asking for or receiving feedback.

Activity 7.2   *Reflection*

Use the chart below to identify the factors that contributed to both the positive and negative feedback experiences you have had in the past. If you can relate your experiences to previous practice experiences, this would be useful; however, you can also look at past work-related performance reviews.

> **My feedback experience was positive because . . .**

> **My feedback experience was negative because . . .**

As this is a reflective activity there is an opportunity to think through your responses and decide on how to approach feedback situations in the future. For example, what would you need to put in place in order to repeat the positive experience? What might you need to alter to ensure the negative experience is not repeated?

As this activity is for your own reflection, there is no outline answer at the end of the chapter.

Activity 7.2 should have demonstrated that there were key areas of each feedback situation that were fundamental to the eventual result. It may be that the negative feedback experience could have been avoided if you had been equipped with additional knowledge and skill in relation to how you could have responded to feedback at the time of the event. Alternatively, Clynes and Raftery (2008) have identified that the preparation of mentors in delivering feedback to students is paramount. If your mentor is lacking the confidence and skill to give fair and accurate feedback, you may have a less than positive experience. Young (2000) cites feedback as a delicate balancing act between fair assessment and protecting vulnerable students. While students value feedback from mentors (Kelly, 2007), mentors are not always prepared for the delivery of feedback (Eraut, 2006). This means that you must not only be prepared for feedback, but also ensure that you are open to receiving feedback by encouraging mentors to do this throughout your practice learning experience.

When should I receive feedback?

You will probably be keen to receive feedback from your mentor through the whole of your practice experience, from the initial interview right through to the final interview. While the literature supports the view that providing feedback to nursing students is imperative (Eaton, 1995), just how and when to do this remains a matter for conjecture. Mentors are advised by the NMC that they essentially have a responsibility to provide students with feedback as often as it is needed to guide performance. As discussed in Chapter 4, the *Standards to Support Learning and Assessment in Practice* reiterate that this is especially important within the context of the sign-off mentor role:

> *Sign-off mentors will require allocated time to ensure that students have effective feedback on their performance so that the ultimate decision on their proficiency is not unexpected. The time allocated may need to be greater earlier in the placement and reduced as they become more confident and competent.*
> (NMC, 2008, p33)

In fact, feedback is an essential aspect of your formative assessment, and it can help you to rate your practice performance more realistically (Glover, 2000). If you are not reaching a competent standard, feedback should be more frequent to provide opportunities to develop and improve. However, your mentor does need to ensure that they are not overdoing your feedback, as you may feel threatened by this. It is essential, therefore, that you have a clear understanding of the two different types of feedback that you may encounter throughout your learning experience in order to prepare for what to do in these situations.

Keeping it casual

Informal feedback occurs randomly throughout a practice experience and is usually given by your mentor in response to a specific event. It can happen at any time and is generally unplanned. It may take place on the spot or as an informal conversation some time later (Eraut, 2006). In general, the earlier that informal feedback becomes routine between a mentor and student during practice experiences, the better. Both you and your mentor will benefit from establishing frequent and spontaneous lines of communication. It is well established that insufficient feedback can impact negatively on your learning experience. Some students have described that the lack of openness of their mentors' feedback increased their anxiety and insecurity during practice (Cahill, 1996). However, if feedback is regularly given on the spot, it can be supportive and constructive and can provide opportunities for reflection (Eraut, 2006).

Mentors also benefit from providing students with regular feedback, as they also gain confidence in discussing your progress. However, you must be very careful not to request continual feedback from your mentor, and it is more than reasonable for them to put some limitations on the amount of feedback you receive. If you do want to receive frequent feedback, you may choose to plan ahead with your mentor for specific time periods when this may be possible. It is also a good idea to put a defined time limit on the discussion (Atkins and Williams, 1995), so that no one becomes frustrated.

Keep in mind that either you or your mentor can instigate feedback and you do not have to wait for your mentor to provide it; in fact, it is in your best interest to request it. Your mentor may volunteer feedback, but if they don't, then ask for it.

Try to use the evidence of learning that you are maintaining in your practice assessment document or portfolio as the basis for feedback. This will help to ensure that your feedback is directly related to the learning outcomes you are attempting and your learning experiences. With a focused feedback event, you will be in a better position to discuss alterations or additions you would like to make to your learning experiences.

Black tie optional

Formal feedback is a planned event and it will normally take place at predetermined stages of your practice experience, namely the initial interview, midpoint review and final interview. It should be structured and ideally be conducted in a quiet area away from the general environment of practice work. Dohrenwend (2002) concludes that privacy and allowing adequate time for what is said to be digested is vital when giving feedback. It should be noted that your mentor is obliged to provide formative feedback on a regular basis (Eraut, 2006). However, some mentors find it particularly difficult to instigate and deliver feedback in a formal setting, partly due to the strong emotional dimension of the interaction (Eraut, 2006). You may also feel vulnerable when receiving feedback (Dohrenwend, 2002), as this is your mentor's opinion of your performance, and will be directly related to the final decision they make for your practice learning outcomes (Sharples, 2007c).

You should be given some time and warning to prepare yourself for the formal feedback event. If you are not given sufficient warning of a formal interview, you may feel quite intimidated and be reluctant to voice your opinions or concerns. A lack of two-way interaction will jeopardise the interaction needed for insight and development (Clynes and Raftery, 2008). To avoid this situation, you should negotiate with your mentor at the start of your practice the dates on which formal feedback in the form of midpoint and final interviews is likely to take place. You can then both feel prepared for these meetings as they will become a routine part of your practice experience.

Once again, part of your preparation for these formal interview situations will involve you having accurate evidence of your learning experiences in your practice assessment document or portfolio. Being able to review all of your experiences will provide the basis for open discussions regarding new learning opportunities or improvements to your current performance.

What feedback should I get?

Regardless of whether you are receiving formal or informal feedback from your mentor, it must always be clear and unambiguous. If you receive too little information, you may be unsure of what is required of you or how this relates to your learning outcomes. On the one hand, when information is withheld, feedback becomes a superficial exercise that lacks the necessary depth to tackle the issues at hand (Dohrenwend, 2002). On the other hand, if feedback includes too much information, you may feel overwhelmed, taking in little of what your mentor has actually said. Clynes and Raftery (2008) comment that feedback should include examples from practice, as well as specific targets and standards. For this reason, Glover (2000) concludes that feedback should be focused on what you can use, rather than the amount your mentor may wish to give.

Case study

Lyn is the mentor to Eunice, who has been with her for some weeks in a special needs school. Eunice has been asked to lead two group therapy sessions but has not shown confidence in delegating tasks to the service users or in managing the timing of the sessions. At the end of the second session Lyn decides to give Eunice some feedback. She feels uncomfortable about this as she does not want Eunice to feel she is being critical. She decides to keep her feedback brief, saying to Eunice, 'I think you need to do some more of those sessions.' Eunice is thrilled. She interprets this feedback as high praise, believing that her mentor wishes her to continue with sessions as she is demonstrating competence. Eunice has no idea that, in actual fact, the feedback was meant to indicate that there was a significant need for improvement. The practice experience continues with Eunice continuing to struggle with group therapy and Lyn frustrated that Eunice is not focusing on the areas she needs to improve.

Activity 7.3   *Reflection*

Consider the events of the case study above. What do you think may eventually happen if Eunice does not receive accurate feedback from her mentor? Try to put yourself in the position of both Lyn and Eunice to reflect on the situation they both face.

As this activity is for your own reflection, there is no outline answer at the end of the chapter.

You will not be able to change behaviour if you do not know what needs to be corrected (Dohrenwend, 2002). Therefore, you cannot and must not rely on assumptions or inferences when you are receiving feedback. For this reason it is vital that, once feedback has been delivered, you clarify what has been said by your mentor in order to rectify any misconceptions. You should remember that the feedback you have heard may not always be the same as the feedback given (Eraut, 2006). In fact, Clynes and Raftery (2008) suggest that students should be encouraged to reflect on their mentor's feedback and outline their interpretation of its content.

No doubt you will have come to this conclusion when you completed Activity 7.3. While Lyn meant no harm, she failed to provide Eunice with the information she required in order to improve. However, as an independent learner, Eunice should also have reflected on the feedback she did receive and ensure that she had grasped the meaning of Lyn's statement. If she had taken this next step of clarifying information, Lyn would have felt more comfortable to explain her concerns and they could have developed a learning plan together aimed at improving Eunice's competence in delegation and time management. As this did not happen, there is little evidence that Eunice will improve her competence in this area.

Constructive feedback

The question of what to discuss and in what way is a constant issue in a feedback situation (Kilbourn, 1990). Within organisational, educational and business domains there has been a great deal of research done into optimum situations and techniques for giving both written and verbal feedback. There is general consensus that constructive feedback is essential and should be frequent (Kilminster et al., 2007), as this will help students to improve their performance (Sharples, 2007c).

A lack of clarity in feedback can have a detrimental effect on the student–mentor relationship and can compromise the self-esteem of both. Your mentor must always ensure that the feedback given is constructive, whether it is delivered formally or informally. This means that it should be objective, non-judgemental and based on specific observations, encouraging discussion and allowing for a positive course to be set for the future (Pearce, 2004). If given appropriately, constructive feedback can boost student confidence, motivation and self-esteem (Baard and Neville, 1996). It is not difficult, therefore, to understand the value of constructive feedback, especially as it supports and encourages learning, motivating students to try again, do better or keep up the good work (Steves, 2005). Likewise, mentors also benefit from providing feedback to students through sharing practice and enhancing learning (Allen, 2002).

Incorporating feedback into your learning cycle

The feedback you receive will make a major difference to your learning experience. On-the-spot feedback from your mentor may typically occur during the learning experiences in which you take part, while informal feedback conversations are more likely to occur during periods of reflection and while you are making sense of your learning experiences. In Figure 7.1, you can see how feedback links with Kolb's experiential learning cycle.

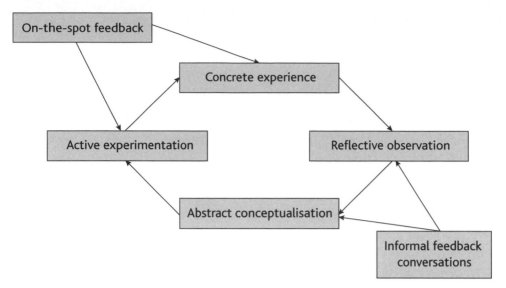

Figure 7.1: Kolb's experiential learning cycle and feedback (adapted from Kolb, 1984, p42)

It is not difficult, therefore, to see the link between feedback and learning in, through and during practice. As feedback on practice performance can be a spontaneous part of the working relationship (Eraut, 2006), it will naturally open the door to your ability and motivation to reflect on your practice. Pugh (1992) argues that the value of a student undertaking self-reflection of their performance cannot be overestimated, as it will provide valuable insight into the student's perception of their own ability. For this reason, self-reflection should be encouraged in feedback situations. Your self-reflection should also provide opportunities for a clear discussion on strengths and weaknesses with your mentor, and help you to regulate your practice experience in a realistic way (Glover, 2000). However, without clarity of feedback, the risk is that you may engage in reflective exercises that are not related to the development of competence (Murphy and Atkins, 1994). If you feel that the feedback you are receiving is not constructive, you should address this with your mentor as soon as possible so that learning opportunities are not lost.

Feedback and self-esteem

You may be quite surprised to find that there is a relationship between feedback and the impact it can have on your self-esteem. While honesty from your mentor is important, you may not interpret the feedback as encouraging if you are emotionally reactive or vulnerable due to low self-esteem (London, 1995). This means that the higher your self-esteem, the more positive your attitude towards assessment in general and, more specifically, towards feedback on performance (Young, 2000). Conversely, if you have low self-esteem, you are more likely to have a fear of negative evaluation (Fleming and Courtney, 1984) and, as a consequence, avoid feedback situations as a coping mechanism (Cahill, 1996). Therefore, while students with high self-esteem may view feedback as an opportunity to improve, those with low self-esteem may adopt a defeatist mentality and perhaps even consider leaving the course (Young, 2000). It is not surprising, therefore, that mentors may also be reluctant to engage in feedback with students because they are uncomfortable in giving what may be interpreted as 'bad news' (Steves, 2005). While it may be obvious that students should be provided with feedback couched in positive terms in order to maintain or improve self-esteem, this does create some difficulty when feedback is required to point out errors or poor performance (Begley and White, 2003).

In earlier chapters we dealt with previous experiences of education as a root cause of negative attitudes and poor self-esteem, especially in your ability to learn. Quite understandably, if you have been exposed to unhappy learning experiences in your past, this baggage will affect your self-esteem. In particular, previous negative experiences may result in you reacting negatively to feedback, as it may be difficult to cast aside past experiences. It is crucially important, therefore, that you ask for feedback that is highly specific (Wiggins, 1998) and related to an evaluation of your behaviour and work performance, so that you do not misinterpret it as an evaluation of your character (Russell, 1994).

Once again, an accurate practice portfolio can assist you and your mentor to establish specific areas for feedback – all of which should be related to your learning experience and their assessment of your competence.

Case study

A student speaks about her experience of receiving feedback during practice.

In my first year of training I had a practice experience in a little community hospital and everyone was really friendly and got on well, and at first I thought it was a really great place to learn. In my second week I was really shocked when my mentor called me aside to say that all the nurses had noticed problems with my documenting in patient charts. I took it really badly and ended up in tears. I couldn't understand why I was being singled out, especially as I was only in first year and they were expecting me to be perfect. I was really angry and I told her I didn't think it was fair that the nurses were all talking about me. She was really quiet for a while and I thought, 'That's got her, she can't defend that one.' She just looked at me and said, 'Would you prefer I said nothing and let you keep making the same mistakes?' I thought about that for ages afterwards, and I realise that she was right; she was only trying to help. I'm in third year now and almost ready to qualify. My current mentor is really impressed with my record keeping and soon I'll be signed off as competent. I might not have made it this far if that mentor in my first year had not been so honest.

There is always a tendency for students with low self-esteem to take any comment as an indictment of themselves (Young, 2000), and if you have had previous negative experiences this can be exacerbated. There is nothing wrong with explaining your feelings about feedback to your mentor, and encouraging them to provide feedback that is specific, focused and emotionally sensitive (Eraut, 2006). If this is taken into consideration, you should be able to view feedback as help and advice, rather than a personal attack.

Documenting feedback

The one area in which you may really struggle is the formal documentation of feedback in your assessment documents. This may be because you may not view feedback positively as a direction for change and instead may interpret it as a definitive judgement on ability (Young, 2000). However, without a written record of an event, there is no evidence to support what has been done or said. The *Standards to Support Learning and Assessment in Practice* conclusively demonstrate the position of the NMC in relation to written feedback:

> *The NMC considers it important that mentors have an audit trail to support their decisions. Throughout a placement where a critical decision on progress is to be made the mentor should ensure that regular feedback is given to the student and that records are kept of guidance given.*
> (NMC, 2008b, p33)

You must understand that, by recording feedback in your assessment document, your mentor is fulfilling a professional obligation. They are accountable and responsible to the NMC for the assessment decision they make about you (NMC, 2008b). This means that the documentation they write must be an accurate record of events. Moreover, the NMC considers documentation to be a vital aspect of the assessment process, as it provides an 'audit trail' to support the decision to pass or fail a student (NMC, 2008b). Mentors have no choice; they are professionally obligated to document the feedback they give to you, as this will provide evidence to support the assessment process and their assessment decision (Sharples, 2007c).

What should my mentor write?

The record of feedback that the mentor writes in your assessment document needs to be both fair and accurate. Written feedback should be dated and signed by you and your mentor, as it often forms the basis of a learning contract or action plan. You should expect the verbal and written feedback you are given to be consistent (Sharples, 2007c), as it should provide an opportunity for setting specific standards and targets (Wiggins, 1998). You can also use the documentation of feedback to discuss your learning needs with other nurses and mentors in your practice area and lecturers from your university.

Don't forget that the feedback you receive from your mentor will require a response from you. This is all part of being an independent learner. You may wish to respond by devising an action plan or perhaps even updating your practice portfolio with additional targets, reflections or objectives. Without taking action on the feedback you receive, it will not be incorporated into your learning experience and will be a wasted opportunity.

Where should my mentor write?

Written feedback should be recorded in the assessment document that the university has provided for you. As previously discussed, there will generally be a section provided within the document for mentors to write their feedback. This will probably be highlighted as initial, midpoint and final interviews. However, additional information is always welcomed by the universities and it is worth finding out where in the assessment document you should advise your mentor to write extra feedback. Your mentor will need to write enough for any concerns or assessment decisions to be explained and for you to be aware of what is required of you in order to improve.

Ongoing achievement records

Since September 2007, the NMC has required that mentors complete an ongoing achievement record for all pre-registration nursing students at the completion of a practice experience (NMC, 2008b). An ongoing achievement record with your mentor's comments must be passed from one practice experience to the next to enable judgements to be made on your progress (NMC, 2008b). This means that the feedback you receive from each practice experience should form part of the discussion that takes place between you and your mentor at each initial interview. In addition, the records that you keep in relation to your practice experiences and evidence of competence will form part of this feedback. The more accurate your feedback records, the more opportunities you will have to develop ongoing practice experiences.

Chapter summary

The feedback you receive from your mentor while you undertake your practice experience is an essential part of your pre-registration learning. This is because feedback provides your mentor with the opportunity of giving you their opinion on your performance. Some mentors struggle with providing feedback, so establishing clear guidelines for how and when feedback will be facilitated is a key aspect of your practice experience. As feedback is based on your mentor's judgement of your competence, it should always be related to the learning outcomes you are trying to achieve. Mentors are professionally obligated to provide students with fair and timely feedback. As we have discovered, it can be particularly challenging to receive feedback if you have low self-esteem, as you are at risk of taking what is said personally. Ideally, feedback should be well timed, well targeted and well said in order to direct growth, motivate and contribute to your learning experience.

Activities: Brief outline answers

Activity 7.1 Johari window exercise (page 96)

This Johari window exercise allowed you not only to develop an understanding of yourself, but also to gain experience in receiving feedback. An example Johari window exercise is given below.

Window 1 – The first window represents facts that you know and others equally know about you. For example, you and your friend both know that your favourite colour is purple.

Window 2 – The second window represents things that you may not know about yourself, but others know about you. For example, you may not realise that you frown when you talk, but your friend recognises this.

Window 3 – The third window represents things that you know about yourself, but others don't know about you. For example, you may have never told your friend that your favourite food is lamb hotpot.

Window 4 – The fourth window represents what you don't yet know about yourself, and your friend doesn't know either. For example, neither of you knows how you might react if you won the lottery. Unless you actually win the lottery, no one will ever know.

In the above example of a Johari window it is possible to see that the shared feedback that takes place in windows 2 and 3 results in unknown elements moving from these windows into window 1, representing shared knowledge. In a practice context, feedback that involves the unknown being known is invaluable in terms of your professional development. Once you become aware of issues that you may need to address, you can begin to structure and plan your learning experiences to achieve learning outcomes. Likewise, the more your mentor understands about your character, the more help they can provide in facilitating appropriate learning opportunities.

Further reading

Eraut, M (2006) Editorial. *Learning in Health and Social Care*, 5(3): 111–18.

This is an easy-to-read article that provides additional insight into the role of feedback and improving work-based performance. Varying types of feedback strategies and tips for constructive communication are discussed.

Useful websites

www.businessballs.com/johariwindowmodel.htm

This website explores the Johari window in some depth, explaining the variations of each window and how feedback can be used to gain insight and open learning experiences.

Chapter 8
Succeeding in practice

Introduction: motivation to learn

Throughout all your practice learning experiences, there will be times when you encounter a variety of issues, problems and obstacles that, if not overcome, will affect the quality of your learning experience. In some cases, the obstacle may be a general lack of motivation. In other circumstances, issues and problems may have a detrimental effect on your learning experience and limit your opportunities for achieving your outcomes.

The first step is to recognise that it is entirely normal to face challenges to your learning while you are in practice. This is not personal to you; the fact is that we do not live in a perfect world and you cannot expect your practice experience to be perfect. The second step is to acknowledge that, in most cases, you can do quite a lot to overcome problems when they occur. Of course, in order to do this you will need to recognise the nature of potential obstacles, and then understand what you can do to either prevent or overcome them. Like all problems, the earlier you address them, the smaller they will be. Therefore, while challenges to your learning are almost impossible to avoid, the good news is that, by facing these issues head-on, you can either avoid these pitfalls altogether, or reduce their impact on your learning experience if and when they occur.

Most student nurses at some point in their pre-registration programme are affected by a reduction in, or complete loss of, motivation. In this chapter we will identify what motivation is and the differences between intrinsic and extrinsic motivation. There will be a focus on the factors that can have a detrimental effect on motivation, including:

- fatigue, tiredness and sleep deprivation due to shift work;
- juggling home and work commitments with practice;
- personality clashes with mentors;
- challenges in learning with a disability.

As each of these issues will affect your ability to learn, we will discuss how you might reduce the stress and anxiety they may induce, in order to succeed during your practice experience.

Let's get motivated

Motivation is one of those strange things – while you cannot actually touch it, feel it, taste it or see it, it really does exist and actually will have one of the biggest roles to play in your learning experience. In fact, you will very often rely heavily on motivation in order to learn – so much so that, without motivation, learning will be almost impossible. The paradox is that, while motivation is essential for learning, you cannot buy motivation, nor can you borrow someone else's. Either you have it or you don't, and someone else telling you to get motivated will have little influence at all.

What is motivation?

Before we go any further, it is important to establish exactly what motivation is in order to understand where it comes from and, more importantly, where it goes when it seems to just disappear.

Activity 8.1   *Reflection*

No doubt you have had times in your life when, one day, you felt very motivated towards doing or achieving something, but the next day the feeling just seems to have vanished. It is worth stopping here and reflecting on this experience and it may help to make some brief notes.

- What were the circumstances of this event?
- Why do you think you felt motivated?
- How long did the motivation last?
- When did your motivation disappear?
- Why do you think you lost motivation?
- What could you have done to prevent loss of motivation?
- If faced with this situation again, what would you do differently?

If you can, try to think of an example from your pre-registration nursing programme during this reflection exercise. This will assist you to put motivation in relation to your learning situation into a current context. If this is not possible, try to reflect on a recent circumstance from your personal life that involved loss of motivation.

An outline of what you might find is given at the end of the chapter.

You will notice that, although you used reflection in Activity 8.1, it is not related to a particular model of reflection. The value of reflection is not related to using a particular model; rather, it is about reviewing your practice and identifying what improvements or alterations are required in future. Reflection is simply a way to learn the most from an experience, and does not always have to be constrained within a formal model.

The frustrating thing about losing motivation is that it is not like losing a set of keys – you can't just hunt around looking for places you might have left it. This does not mean that, if you lose motivation, it can't be found again; it simply means that motivation is not a tangible object that can be physically picked up or put down. In its simplest form, motivation may be defined as the forces or processes that cause individuals to act in a specific way (Maitland, 1995). However, motivation as a theory and as a method of explaining human behaviour cannot be limited to, or explained through, just one definition. The problem, of course, as Vernon (1969) explains, is that motivation is such an internal experience that it remains difficult to classify, define or interpret. Despite these difficulties, many notable theorists have attempted to, and indeed continue to, interpret and promote our understanding of human motivation.

Maslow's hierarchy of needs

One such theorist was Abraham Maslow, a behavioural scientist who developed a theory about the rank and satisfaction of various human needs. This is widely referred to today as **Maslow's hierarchy of needs**. Maslow (1943) based his motivational theory on the concept that the integrated wholeness of the organism must be one of the foundation stones of human motivation. In other words, your motivation is directly related to who you are, your personality and 'what makes you tick'. His theory of motivation proposed that all individuals have a set hierarchy of needs that they have a desire to satisfy (Maitland, 1995). In addition, Maslow (1943) argued that humans need to arrange themselves in hierarchies, where the appearance of one need rests on the prior satisfaction of others. The order of these needs is represented in Figure 8.1.

It is quite easy to see that, in order of needs, motivation begins with the satisfaction of physiological needs and progresses in turn through needs related to safety, belongingness and love, esteem and self-actualisation (Maslow, 1987). In its simplest form, Maitland (1995) suggests that Maslow's motivational theory allows individuals to move up through the various levels of the hierarchical pyramid once these classified needs are developed, satisfied and fulfilled at each level.

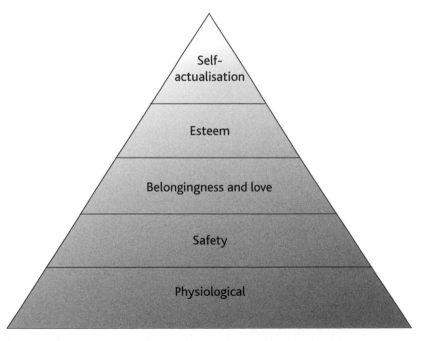

Figure 8.1: Maslow's hierarchy of needs (adapted from Maslow, 1987, pp15–22)

Learning and motivation

Has it ever occurred to you that, by undertaking your nursing training, you are striving for the top two levels of the pyramid? The act of learning, increasing your knowledge, is associated with a need for esteem and self-actualisation. This is great news and you should rightly be proud of yourself for wanting to attain these levels. However, it is not difficult to see that the higher up the pyramid you go, the greater risk there is that something at a lower stage may impact on your higher-order motivation. In fact, many student nurses feel that Murphy's Law – 'If it can go wrong, it will go wrong' – was written especially for them.

Activity 8.2 — *Critical thinking*

Each stage of Maslow's hierarchy of needs represents a range of different needs. The premise is that we need to feel fulfilled at each stage before the next stage of the motivational pyramid can be reached. Have a look at the examples below to see the types of needs that are represented at each stage.

Self-actualisation	Confidence, achievement, personal growth, fulfilment
Esteem	Recognition, reputation, dignity, status
Belongingness and love	Family, friends, partner, children
Safety	Job security, shelter, health
Physiological	Food, water, air, warmth, sleep

Take some time to refer back to the notes you made in Activity 8.1. Try to identify where you were on the motivational pyramid when you felt motivated. What 'need' were you satisfying while you were at this level? Now look at the categories below this level. Can you identify a change in your circumstances that may have influenced your motivation? Perhaps you were at the esteem level when something happened to change your feeling of safety. If this was the case, you would have quickly lost motivation for improving your esteem and focused on re-establishing your safety.

Take your time in matching your circumstances with the levels of the pyramid, as this will help you critically to analyse the situation. Not only will you gain insight into what happened, but also why it happened. This is your opportunity to begin understanding more about yourself in relation to the strength of your motivational drivers for undertaking the pre-registration course, and how this motivation may be influenced by other factors in your personal circumstances.

An outline of what you might find is given at the end of the chapter.

It is quite easy to see how physiological needs are the priority in the motivational pyramid. Our most basic needs in life are those that keep us alive and, if these are at risk, it is not difficult to understand that there would be little motivation to move on to the next stage of the pyramid. This isn't to say that all examples of needs must be met, but we must feel secure and happy at each level before we can move on. In fact, pivotal to Maslow's motivational theory is his belief that any motivated behaviour is a channel through which many basic needs may simultaneously be expressed or satisfied (Maslow, 1943). In other words, your motivation to do or not do something is rarely down to just one factor. A whole range of influences will contribute to your overall motivation, and these can occur at any stage of the motivational pyramid. This also means that your motivation will be influenced by a combination of needs that contribute to your personality.

Scenario

Sarah works for a multinational insurance firm and has spent many years building up her reputation and progressing within the organisation. Her dream is to become the managing director of the company and she has spent her entire career working towards this ultimate goal. She is informed that a new post is being developed and she spends days preparing for the interview, as this will be one more stepping stone towards her ultimate goal. On the day of the interview Sarah's partner becomes very ill and is rushed to hospital. Within seconds, all Sarah's motivation for the new job and personal ambition disappears. Her priority changes instantly, from promoting her own need for esteem to protecting her need for belongingness and love. It is only once she is assured that her partner will make a full recovery that she can once again concentrate on, and motivate herself towards, personal ambitions.

Like all skills, developing ways to motivate yourself for learning will require some practice. Your nursing course should have already provided you with some skills for planning your practice learning, for example interpersonal, communication, decision-making, negotiation and problem-solving skills. These are all assets that you can use in order to motivate yourself during practice learning experiences. However, as Sharples et al. (2007) recognise, it is naive to assume that all nursing students entering the practice environment will automatically acquire the knowledge, skills and attitude to be successful. It may well be that motivation is missing. If you are currently lacking motivation for practice learning, you must rectify this.

Intrinsic and extrinsic motivation

We have already established that motivation is strongly related to events that happen around you and also your personality. Obviously, there will be events that take place outside your control that will ultimately affect your motivation. However, in some instances you can change or predict the practice events that may affect your motivation and, in doing so, protect the quality of your learning experience. It is important to recognise, however, that while a loss of motivation during a practice experience will rarely mean the end of the experience, it will usually signify a loss of interest in learning. If you happen to be undertaking your practice experience with no interest in learning, there is little point being there.

Motivation is your responsibility

While it is not difficult to understand that seizing learning opportunities will be important to your practice experience, having the motivation to do this is an entirely different matter. The reason for this may be related to the origin of your motivation. Is your motivation intrinsic or extrinsic? **Intrinsic motivation** is generally considered to be associated with achieving a goal or performing a task for its own sake. In contrast, **extrinsic motivation** stems from a desire for reward (Benabou and Tirole, 2003). In most cases you will find that both types will contribute to your overall motivation during practice experiences and there is no problem with this. However, you will run into difficulties if you depend entirely on extrinsic motivational forces, as these can fluctuate and dissipate very quickly. If you rely on being rewarded as a means of generating your motivation, what will happen if the rewards stop or are not as frequent as you would like? Obviously, your motivation will also suffer. It may be, then, that your motivation for seeking out and engaging with learning experiences wanes because it is rooted in extrinsic motivational forces rather than grounded in intrinsic aspects of your personality.

A key aspect of maintaining your motivation to learn is through understanding and accepting that your motivation is intrinsic to you. In other words, you will need to accept your own responsibility for learning in, through and during practice (Elcock et al., 2007). In order to fulfil your learning plan, you will need to be motivated enough to negotiate your learning needs throughout the practice experience (Begley and Brady, 2002). If you are dependent on extrinsic forces for motivation, the likelihood is that you will be unable to shift from task-based activities to a holistic model of learning (Spouse, 2003). If you are not motivated to learn, it is very unlikely that anyone, especially your mentor, will be motivated to stimulate your learning for you.

You may well find that you begin a practice experience feeling motivated; however, as time progresses your motivation decreases to the point where you stop being focused on your learning experiences and instead begin to focus on factors such as how long it is until the end and what grade you may achieve. Unless you stay focused on learning throughout the entirety of the practice experience, you risk losing all intrinsic motivation to learn and instead will focus all your motivation on extrinsic aspects of reward. Your vision of success will be based on irrelevant factors such as completing the required number of weeks, rather than on learning experience and developing competence.

Success and motivation

It should now be possible to understand that motivation plays a very significant role in your opportunities for, and experience of, learning in practice. Success during a practice experience should never be viewed as a given, and while you may be provided with mentor support and an opportunity for practice learning, ultimately it is you who must take responsibility for your own practice learning experience. To succeed during a practice experience you must take full advantage of your supernumerary status (Elcock et al., 2007). If you do not have the motivation to do this, you will not make the most of your practice learning opportunities. Your success during practice experience will require that you continually plan and revise your learning opportunities and are motivated to negotiate additional learning experiences (Elcock, 2006).

Types of motivation

The following clarifies the main differences between intrinsic and extrinsic motivational factors that may influence your practice learning experience.

Extrinsic motivation:

- positive feedback from a mentor;
- passing a practice experience;
- praise from a patient or client;
- admiration from family or friends.

Intrinsic motivation:

- an overall desire to learn;
- wanting to increase your own knowledge and skill;
- learning from your mistakes;
- developing your professional role.

The difference between the two types of motivation should be very clear: extrinsic motivation tends to be associated with short-term rewards, whereas intrinsic motivation tends to be associated with long-term goals or aspirations. While there is nothing wrong with having extrinsic factors within your motivational drivers, there must also be some element of intrinsic motivation to counterbalance this when extrinsic factors are limited.

Activity 8.3 — *Reflection*

Take the time now to make a list of the things that you rely on to motivate you during your practice experiences. You may like to reflect on a previous specific experience of being in practice as a reference point for your ideas. Separate your motivation during this experience into extrinsic and intrinsic factors.

Extrinsic motivation	Intrinsic motivation

In particular, think about the rewards that you may rely on for your extrinsic motivation.

continued opposite . . .

---

continued . . .

- Do you require these hourly, daily or weekly to sustain motivation?
- What happens if you do not get the rewards you require?
- Do you have intrinsic motivation that you can refer back to and rely on if extrinsic motivation does not take place?

As this activity is for your own reflection, there is no outline answer at the end of the chapter.

Why do I lose motivation?

The reason that you may lose motivation during a practice experience will be very personal to you. However, if you do tend to lose motivation, you may find that your core motivational drivers are heavily dependent on extrinsic factors. You will need to develop some intrinsic drivers to cover the periods when extrinsic factors diminish. If you can't think of any intrinsic factors, you may need to think about the fundamental reason that you embarked on a career in nursing in the first place. Did you begin this journey with intrinsic motivation? If so, these initial reasons and feelings should be far more solid and reliable than any extrinsic motivational drivers – and they will need to be. They will need to sustain you through a variety of different learning experiences.

Case study

A former student speaks about her motivation to complete her nursing course.

I'm not really sure why I wanted to be a nurse. I guess I just fell into it. There was a lot of pressure from home to do something when I finished college and I had a friend who was doing nursing so I sort of thought, why not? It was OK for a while, but then I had this really difficult placement; I had to travel a long way, I was always tired and I had all this pressure with theory assignments due in. I seriously thought about quitting, I just couldn't see much point in going on. Luckily for me, I came to my senses and realised that it wouldn't always be this bad and if I hung in there it could be a career for life. I'm two years qualified now and I can honestly say that I love my work; not a day goes by when I don't learn something new. I'm even off to work as a nurse in Australia for a year. If I had given up that just wouldn't be possible.

Success in practice learning

Let's start by looking at what it really means to succeed during a practice experience. Success will have the following attributes.

- Learning outcomes are matched with learning experiences throughout the practice experience.
- Learning experiences are agreed with your mentor and reviewed regularly throughout the practice experience.
- Learning plans that support the learning experiences are followed and kept under regular review.
- There are frequent opportunities for reflection and feedback related to learning experiences.
- Formal interviews are timely and focused on improving the learning experience and achieving outcomes.
- A practice portfolio is maintained that provides evidence of learning experiences and achievement of outcomes.

It should be clear from this list that the success of a practice experience is based on the value of the learning experience. If all these factors are in place, you should be able to achieve all your learning outcomes. Conversely, if your learning experience in practice is compromised in any way, the experience will not be successful and learning outcomes may not be achieved.

Obstacles to success

There are several key obstacles that could impact on the success of your learning experience in practice. If these obstacles are not dealt with, your motivation may also be compromised. The factors that can limit success could include:

- general fatigue;
- sleep deprivation;
- financial concerns;
- caring for dependants in your personal life;
- supporting family and friends;
- personality clashes;
- a disability that impacts on learning.

If you are facing obstacles to success, you must not ignore these issues. Unless you address your own barriers, you will not be able to seize all the learning opportunities available as a result of your supernumerary role.

Sleep, fatigue and learning

If you undertake your practice experiences feeling fatigued, you will find it very difficult to succeed. Your motivation for learning and contributing fully to your learning experiences will be severely compromised. If you refer back to Activity 8.2, you will see that sleep forms one of the most basic physiological needs. If you are not getting enough rest, chronic fatigue will result. It is well established that shift work is notorious for interrupting sleep patterns and contributing to sleep deprivation. Anecdotally, many nurses report that working the night shift and adjusting to sleeping during the day causes the most stress. As a result, many shift workers exist in a constant state of sleep deprivation (Stryjewski et al., 2002). The NMC requires you, as a pre-registration student nurse, to participate in the full range of 24/7 shifts (NMC, 2004). By default this means that you will need to undertake shift work as a part of your learning experience, and participate in a combination of early, late and night shifts. While this is primarily designed to give students insight into the needs of their patients during a full 24-hour day, sleep deprivation due to shift work may cause you to lose motivation to learn. To succeed in practice learning you will need to 'learn' how to cope with shift work.

Tips for surviving shift work

- Avoid caffeinated drinks after midnight. While they may help to keep you awake during the night, they also make it difficult to sleep the next morning.
- Wear sunglasses home from work, even on a cloudy day. The reduced light may help convince your brain that it is night.
- Sleep in a cool room. Body temperature drops at night, so it helps to recreate this coolness when trying to sleep during the day.
- If you like to watch television before bed, record a programme from the night before. It may help to trick your brain into thinking it is night-time.
- Invest in blackout curtains and earplugs. Too much light and noise will stimulate your brain and prevent restful sleep.

Source: Adapted from Sharples and Kelly (2006)

Home, family and learning

There can be no doubt that your home, family and social life will be impacted by your nurse training, especially during practice experiences. Almost without exception, your family and social life will be at the mercy of a rolling series of late, early and weekend shifts (Sharples, 2006). No matter how prepared you are, the reality is that, once in practice, your motivation may well suffer if the terms of your practice experience are having a negative impact on those you love. Sometimes, no matter how well planned and thought out your practice experiences are, there may be times when this will happen.

While everyone has very different personal circumstances, there are some key areas of social and personal lives that are commonly affected because of practice experiences. These can include the following.

- Financial pressures – the requirement to be flexible for practice experiences makes permanent part-time employment impossible. Means-tested grants do not always financially compensate for loss of regular employment.
- Interruptions to family and social life – you can no longer expect set days off, and may miss out on regular family and social events during practice experiences.

- Caring for dependants – your practice experience may impact on taking children to school or collecting them, and may result in costly childcare.

Have another look at Activity 8.2 and you will see that these factors fit in with your fundamental need for belongingness and love. If this is threatened during your practice experience, the result will be a loss of, or reduction in, motivation to learn. In reality, solutions for these problems can be very difficult. You will need to accept that your practice experiences will affect your social and family life, so you will need to have a plan for how to cope with this before the practice experience begins (Sharples, 2006). You may also need to accept that, where difficulties are outside your control or cannot be resolved, you may need to take a break in your programme until such time as the issue or problem has been dealt with. If you are having ongoing problems within your home and family life that are impacting on your practice experience, these will take precedence, and no amount of intrinsic motivation will override these difficulties.

Case study

Wendy has always wanted a career in nursing and decides that, when her youngest child reaches school age, she will commence her training. She is a single parent and has made arrangements for her sister to care for her two children during evening, night and weekend shifts while she is undertaking her practice experience. During her first year of training this arrangement suits everybody; her children are well cared for by their aunt, and Wendy can concentrate on her studies. However, in her second year of training Wendy's sister becomes ill and can no longer care for the children. Wendy tries to make alternative arrangements; however, she cannot afford after-school childcare and her children are unhappy being cared for by different friends every day. As she has no options for night or weekend care, Wendy cannot commit to the practice area rota and is forced to take sick leave on these shifts. The last thing on Wendy's mind, when she is able to be in practice, is learning from the experience, as she has lost all motivation. She has no option but to take a break from the programme and she defers for six months. During this time, she is able to care for her sister and she no longer feels stressed as her children are happy. At the end of the six months, Wendy's sister is fully recovered and is able to resume caring for the children. Wendy is able to return to her training at the point she left, fully committed and focused on her learning.

Personality clashes and learning

No matter how motivated you are before a practice experience, this can soon diminish if you clash personalities with your mentor. Just as there are no perfect mentors, there are no perfect students, so from time to time personality clashes will occur. Clashes can occur for any number of reasons and it would be rare to find that there is not some level of fault on both sides. This is not to say that nothing can be done to reduce or eradicate personality clashes, as there is a range of solutions to these types of problems. However, it does need to be understood that personality clashes are almost impossible to prevent, and at some point you will no doubt have a clash of personalities with a mentor.

Some of the more common reasons for personality clashes include:

- the mentor and student having a difference of opinion related to the shift rota;
- the mentor or student not liking the way the other person speaks to them;
- the mentor or student using body language that is viewed as offensive;
- either mentor or student showing a lack of interest;
- the mentor and student having a different opinion regarding roles and responsibilities.

If you already have some experience of practice, some of these circumstances may be quite familiar.

However, a personality clash is to do with personalities only. It does not cover any failings of your mentor in terms of their professional accountability and responsibility. These issues have been dealt with extensively in Chapter 4. If you feel that your mentor is not fulfilling their role, this should be raised with someone senior in the practice area or a support lecturer from your university. A personality clash is separate from these types of issues and is simply a failure of two individuals to get along, rather than a failure in mentorship requirements.

A personality clash alone is not enough to justify a change of mentor. To change mentors just because you are not getting along resolves nothing, and only serves to avoid a situation that has the potential to be resolved. This is not to say that a personality clash should be trivialised, as a successful practice experience will be compromised if you are not getting along with your mentor. However, putting this into some perspective, it is not reasonable to assume that you will be able to avoid personality clashes simply because they are difficult. What will you do if you do not particularly like the personality of your patients? Is it reasonable that you will be able to avoid patients you don't like, or who don't like you? The answer, of course, is a definite 'No'. This means that you will need to try to resolve personality clashes with mentors, as in doing so you will also be learning valuable skills of communication and negotiation.

The good news is that it is possible to resolve personality clashes. Have a look again at Chapter 7 and the Johari window in Activity 7.1 on page 96. The second window represents what we may not know about ourselves, but others know about us. So, there may be aspects of your character or personality that can annoy or irritate others. You will have no way of knowing what it is about your personality that a mentor may find irritating before you meet them, just as they will have no idea what you may dislike about them.

Case study

A mentor speaks about resolving a personality clash with a student.

A few years ago I was mentoring a student in the mental health resources centre. We were always polite to each other and I didn't think there were any problems, but one day she asked to speak to me and I could see she was really upset. Then she tells me that it really upsets her when I ignore her in the morning. I explained that I'm not a morning person and I don't really like chatting in the morning, not until I've had a

continued overleaf . . .

continued . . . .

> coffee anyway. I hadn't even realised I was ignoring her and felt really guilty when she pointed it out. We had a good laugh about it and the next day she even brought us both a latte. We had no more problems after that; we just needed to talk it through. Actually, I'm glad she pointed it out. I make a real effort now every morning not to be grumpy, which I'm sure everyone appreciates.

In some cases the personality clash you experience may be related to the fact that your mentor has a very different learning style from yours. Perhaps you are a reflector by nature in your learning approach. If your mentor is more of an activist, this can lead to conflict and misunderstandings. Your mentor may misinterpret your preference for reflecting before acting as laziness or boredom. You, in turn, may misinterpret their desire for you to become more involved in activities as pushiness. Yet, whatever the reason, the only way you will be able to understand the origin of the personality clash is through communication. Remember, you don't have to become best friends with your mentor; you just need to find a way to work and learn together without conflict. If you fail to resolve these conflicts, your motivation for learning in practice will be compromised.

Disability and learning

If you are a pre-registration student nurse with a disability, your disability does not mean you cannot succeed on your pre-registration programme. Nor does it mean that you will automatically succeed on your pre-registration programme. What your disability does ensure is the following:

> *Programme providers should consider how reasonable adjustments could be made to ensure that disabled applicants can fully participate in the theory and practice aspects of the programme without compromising safety.*
> (NMC, 2010, p10)

In other words, your disability will be taken into account in order to ensure that you are able to undertake the nursing programme. If you meet the entry criteria for your pre-registration programme, you are legally entitled to undertake each element of your course without discrimination. In other words, your disability cannot be used as a reason to either include or exclude you from commencing your nursing study. However, your entitlement to undertake a course does not, and should never be mistaken for, an entitlement for passing the course of study. Your disability is not a free ticket for passing. If you do not achieve your learning outcomes during a practice experience, this would not be seen as discriminatory. Discrimination in this context would only exist if your university or practice area did not make reasonable adjustments for your disability to ensure fairness and equality (DDA, 2005).

What do we mean by disability?

In 1995, the Disability Discrimination Act (DDA) was introduced into legislation with the intention of protecting the rights of those with disabilities. According to the Act, it an offence to discriminate against an individual because of their disability (DDA, 1995). Within this Act a disability was classed as:

- a mental or physical impairment that has an adverse effect on the ability to carry out normal day-to-day activities;
- [and where] the adverse effect is substantial and long-term, meaning it has lasted for 12 months or is likely to last for 12 months more.

Since the original DDA 1995, there have been several amendments to the Act that have relevance within nursing, and particularly nursing and midwifery education. These include:

- 1995 Disability Discrimination Act;
- 2001 Special Educational Needs and Disability Act;
- 2004 Amendment to Disability Discrimination Act 1995;
- 2005 Disability Discrimination Act.

The sum total of all these various Acts of Parliament is that a person with a disability should not be excluded from an educational opportunity as a result of that disability. In particular, the 2001 Special Educational Needs and Disability Act makes it unlawful for a disabled student to be excluded from a university course or programme because of their disability if they meet the entry requirements and if professional/academic standards can be maintained.

In addition, the 2004 amendment to the DDA 1995 puts a duty on practice providers to make reasonable adjustments for disabled students, and to this end the NMC has been required to ensure that the competency standards for entry to the professional register are objectively justifiable.

Finally, the DDA 2005 states that all publicly funded bodies (i.e. universities) are required to provide a disability scheme for the promotion and implementation of disability equality in their organisation.

As many nursing students choose to disclose their disability on entry to the pre-registration programme, we can see the different types of disability that students are living with. These include:

- learning disabilities;
- visual disabilities;
- hearing disabilities;
- mobility disabilities;
- mental health disabilities;
- long-term health conditions.

For each of these disabilities your university and practice area would be required to consider any reasonable adjustments that may be required.

What are reasonable adjustments?

A reasonable adjustment is something that a university or practice area might reasonably be expected to do in order to ensure that your disability is not preventing you from undertaking learning experiences. You can expect that adjustments will be made to ensure that you are not discriminated against during your practice experience, although you should not expect to achieve your learning outcomes successfully without demonstrating the necessary level of competence. For disabled students, this can mean that your practice experience can be a daunting and challenging experience. You may need to overcome a number of obstacles related to your disability in order to succeed. This may in turn affect your motivation.

Confidentiality and self-disclosure of your disability

There is no law that says that you must disclose your disability to anyone during the course of your nursing programme. This includes your mentor during your practice experience. Such information is classified as sensitive personal information and is covered by the Data Protection Act 1998. For this same reason, your university is not legally allowed to notify the practice area of your disability, nor do you have to disclose this information to the university. However, if you have chosen not to disclose your disability, the university is under no obligation to make reasonable adjustments that may ordinarily apply to your disability. Likewise, your mentor in practice and the practice provider are under no legal obligation to make reasonable adjustments if you do not make them aware of your disability. This means that the only way a mentor can know of your disability is if you tell them.

Case study

Rachel is about to commence her practice experience. She has recently been assessed and diagnosed as having dyslexia. So far, she has chosen not to disclose her disability for fear of being labelled. During school years Rachel was often ridiculed for being slow and she doesn't want the same treatment from her mentor. Much to Rachel's surprise, she discovers that her mentor also has dyslexia, and she realises that, in disclosing her disability, she is able to access help from her university. If Rachel had chosen not to inform her mentor of her disability, additional help and support would not have been available. Rachel has a great practice experience; the help she receives reduces her anxiety and allows her to maintain motivation.

First, Rachel is provided with clear yellow overlays that she can place over written material to help with reading. In addition, the university provides Rachel with access to a laptop so that she can write her practice portfolio easily and delete mistakes quickly. Finally, Rachel's mentor recommends that she carry a notebook with her and write in unfamiliar words so that she can practise spelling. These small adjustments ensure that Rachel can stop struggling with her disability and instead focus on all her learning experiences.

The role of my mentor

If you do choose to disclose your disability, help will be made available to you. This is the law, and there is legislation to protect your rights and prevent discrimination. Some of the help you receive in relation to your disability will be channelled via your mentor. It should be pointed out, however, that your mentor is not automatically required to know the exact nature of the reasonable adjustments that may be required for each student with a disability, or your special circumstances. In order to assist you in their role, the *Standards to Support Learning and Assessment in Practice* (NMC, 2008b) require that your mentor must be provided with university support to ensure that they fulfil their professional and legal obligation in mentoring a student with a disability. However, once the reasonable adjustments are made clear, your mentor is required to facilitate these adjustments.

What if I don't succeed?

Despite all your best efforts, you may not be successful in achieving all of your learning outcomes during a practice experience. While this is obviously disappointing, there is no need to view yourself as a failure if this happens. Initially, you should take some time to assess why this has happened so that you can ensure that you put measures in place to rectify the situation. You will be offered a second attempt at any practice experience where you have not been successful at the first attempt, so you will need to ensure that you make the most of your second opportunity. In particular, you should review your preparation for the practice experience, and also review learning plans and experiences, the quality of your practice portfolio as evidence of competence and your attitude to constructive feedback. It's sometimes useful to think of what you would do differently if you had your time over again. An honest review of your practice experience can help to identify the issues that you may need to address on the second attempt.

Help from your mentor

If you are facing a second attempt of a practice experience, it is very important that you receive very clear feedback from your mentor on the areas in which you need to improve. The best way to achieve this is to have very detailed feedback written within your ongoing achievement record. This will ensure that you can discuss this information with your next mentor and develop focused learning plans. In addition, you will be able to refer to this information throughout your next practice experience without relying solely on your memory.

Chapter summary

Throughout all your practice experiences there will be times when you are faced with obstacles that have the potential to impact on your learning. Unless you can overcome these obstacles, your motivation to take full advantage of your supernumerary role and engage with all learning experiences will be compromised. The success of your learning experience will depend on you developing both intrinsic and extrinsic motivational drivers. These will need to sustain you through a wide variety of challenges, be it coping with the demands of shift work or juggling your home and family life around the structure of practice experiences. In addition, there will be personal issues that arise, personality clashes and/or coping with a disability. The good news is that, no matter what the challenges, there are practical solutions that you can develop to override the difficulties. By using these strategies you can maintain motivation to learn in, through and during your practice experience.

Activities: Brief outline answers

Activity 8.1 Motivation (page 109)

- **What were the circumstances of this event?** You were required to prepare for an OSCE examination. You may have felt very motivated in the beginning, perhaps even visiting the simulation labs to practise skills outside class time. Over time, however, the motivation decreased, to the point where you stopped practising altogether, even missing scheduled classes. The OSCE examination goes very badly and you do not achieve your outcomes.
- **Why do you think you felt motivated?** Everyone in the class was originally saying they were going to practise in the simulation labs and you became excited by their enthusiasm.
- **How long did the motivation last?** The motivation lasted for about two weeks.
- **When did your motivation disappear?** You stopped feeling motivated one month before the OSCE examination and in the last three weeks you stopped practising independently and also missed the class.
- **Why do you think you lost motivation?** You were only motivated in the beginning because other people said they would practise also, and you were part of a big group. By the second week only three other people were still going to extra practice sessions and, on the last occasion you went, you were there by yourself.
- **What could you have done to prevent loss of motivation?** You could have encouraged more people to keep practising with you, as you recognise that you find it easier to keep motivated if you are not feeling isolated. You also lost motivation as it's impossible to practise some scenarios alone. This may have involved setting up an online discussion board or texting everyone with details of practice times, perhaps even suggesting a trip to a coffee house afterwards to get everyone motivated and improve morale. If this didn't work, you could have found out if there were other classes to join for extra practice sessions.
- **If faced with this situation again, what would you do differently?** I would try to do all of the things that help me to stay motivated by organising a more structured approach. Maybe I could post a schedule of extra practice times on our virtual notice board, and suggest that people pair up so that no one feels as if they are practising alone. In future, I'm not going to let a loss of motivation stand in the way of my success.

Activity 8.2 Maslow's hierarchy of needs (page 111)

Your original motivation in wanting to attend additional simulation sessions is related to your need for self-actualisation. You want to do well in your exams, achieve a high grade and feel confident in practice situations. However, you also have a very strong need for love and belongingness. In this situation you need friends who will support you during simulation sessions. Without the support of even one friend you feel lonely and isolated, and very quickly lose motivation to achieve your personal goals. You realise that, in order to keep motivated in the simulation lab, you will need to ensure that you are part of a class or have at least one friend to practise with.

Further reading

Disability Discrimination Act (DDA) (2005) Available online at **www.legislation.gov.uk/ukpga/2005/13/contents**.

The full act explains in detail the current legislation related to disability in the UK and implications for the public and private sector.

Useful websites

www.equalityhumanrights.com

This is a useful website for current information about rights in different settings.

www.legislation.gov.uk

This website contains all UK Parliament Public General Acts from 1988 onwards, including all disability discrimination acts.

Glossary

Andragogical: a broad term that is used to describe learning strategies focused on how adults learn; it can also refer to the processes that are used to engage adult learners in the structure of the learning experience.

Care pathways: an outline of anticipated care that, when placed in an appropriate timeframe, helps patients to progress through planned treatment.

Experiential learning: the process of making meaning and thereby learning through direct experiences.

Extrinsic motivation: a desire to improve, or to achieve or attain a goal that is related to a specific reward.

Fitness for practice: an expectation by the NMC that, at the point of qualification, nurses must be able to relate to the changing needs of the health services and the communities that they serve, responding to current and future need in terms of provision of care, management of care, a health-for-all orientation and lifelong learning.

High-road transfer: the non-automatic examination of a situation with the aim of generating an alternative action when faced with an unfamiliar task.

Intrinsic motivation: an internal desire to improve, or to achieve or attain a goal.

Knowledgeable doer: a student who, after pre-registration education, should be able, on registration, to apply knowledge, understanding and skills when performing to the standards required in employment.

Low-road transfer: skills that have been developed and can be used automatically with little conscious deliberation.

Maslow's hierarchy of needs: a predetermined group of motivating factors developed by Abraham Maslow, listed in order and levels of importance.

Mentor: a registrant who has met the requirements of the NMC mentorship standard and is responsible and accountable for facilitating learning and assessing competence of students in a practice setting.

Motivation: the reasons and/or principles behind why humans act, respond or perform in certain ways, including the drivers for making decisions.

Reflection: Examination of personal thoughts or actions to assist with development of future personal and professional competencies.

Rostered service: the final 20 per cent of practice learning time spent, prior to 1999, by pre-registration students; for the first 80 per cent, they had supernumerary status.

Self-direction: an approach that relies heavily on students being responsible for their own learning; components can include distance programmes, blended learning, learning logs, learning contracts or problem-based packages.

Self-regulation: an individual's ability to attain personalised academic goals through the use of proactive, self-directed internal and external strategies.

Sign-off mentor: an appropriately qualified nurse, midwife or health visitor who signs off students at the final assessment of practice, and confirms to the NMC that the required competencies for entry to the register have been achieved.

Supernumerary status: in relation to students, this means that they shall not, as part of their programme of preparation, be employed by any persons or body under a contract of service to provide nursing care; students are considered to be additional to the workforce requirements and staffing establishment figures.

References

Allen, C (2002) Peers and partners: a stakeholder evaluation of preceptorship in mental health nursing. *Nurse Researcher*, 9(3): 68–84.

Andrews, M and Roberts, D (2003) Supporting student nurses learning in and through clinical practice: the role of the clinical guide. *Nurse Education Today*, 23: 474–81.

Aston, L and Molassiotis, A (2003) Supervising and supporting student nurses in clinical placements: the peer support intuitive. *Nurse Education Today*, 23: 202–10.

Atkins, S and Williams, A (1995) Registered nurses' experiences and mentoring undergraduate nursing students. *Journal of Advanced Nursing*, 21: 1006–15.

Baard, P and Neville, S (1996) The intrinsically motivated nurse: help and hindrance from evaluation feedback sessions. *Journal of Nursing Administration*, 26(7/8): 19–26.

Beck, C (1993) Nursing students' initial clinical experience: a phenomenological study. *International Journal of Nursing Studies*, 30(6): 489–97.

Begley, C and Brady, A (2002) Irish diploma in nursing students' first clinical allocation: the views of nurse managers. *Journal of Nursing Management*, 10: 339–47.

Begley, C and White, P (2003) Irish nursing students' changing self-esteem and fear of negative evaluation during their preregistration programme. *Journal of Advanced Nursing*, 42(4): 390–401.

Benabou, R and Tirole, J (2003) Intrinsic and extrinsic motivation. *Review of Economic Studies*, 70: 489–520.

Boud, D, Cohen, R and Walker, D (1993) *Using Experience for Learning.* Buckingham: The Society for Research into Higher Education and Open University Press.

Cahill, H (1996) A qualitative analysis of student nurses' experiences of mentorship. *Journal of Advanced Nursing*, 24: 791–9.

Cantor, J (1995) *Experiential Learning in Higher Education.* Washington, DC: The George Washington University.

Carroll, M, Curtis, L, Higgins, A, Nicholl, H, Redmond, R and Timmins, F (2001) Is there a place for reflective practice in the nursing curriculum? *Nurse Education in Practice*, 2: 13–20.

Chambers, M (1998) Some issues in the assessment of clinical practice: a review of the literature. *Journal of Clinical Nursing*, 7(3): 201–8.

Clynes, M (2008) Providing feedback on clinical performance to student nurses in children's nursing: challenges facing preceptors. *Journal of Children's and Young People's Nursing*, 2(1): 29–35.

Clynes, M and Raftery, S (2008) Feedback: an essential element of student learning in clinical practice. *Nurse Education in Practice*, 8(6): 405–11.

Corder, N (2008) *Learning to Teach Adults: An introduction*, 2nd edition. London: Routledge.

Crawford, D (2004) The role of aging in adult learning: implications for instructors in higher education. *New Horizons for Learning.* Available online at www.marthalakecov.org/~building/lifelong/higher_ed/crawford.htm (accessed 20 March 2011).

Davies, B, Neary, M and Phillips, R (1994) *The Practitioner-Teacher.* Cardiff: School of Education, University of Wales.

Dawson, C (2006) *The Mature Student's Study Guide.* Oxford: How To Books.

Delahaye, B and Ehrich, L (2008) Complex learning preferences and strategies of older adults. *Educational Gerontology*, 34(8): 649–62.

Dennison, B and Kirk, R (1990) *Do, Review, Learn, Apply: A simple guide to experiential learning.* Oxford: Blackwell Education.

Dewey, J (1933*) How We Think: A restatement of the relation of reflective thinking to the educative process.* New York: Heath and Co.

Disability Discrimination Act (DDA) (1995) Available online at www.legislation.gov.uk/ukpga/1995/50/contents (accessed 20 March 2011).

Disability Discrimination Act (DDA) (1995) (Amendment 2004) Available online at www.opsi.gov.uk.si/si2003/draft/20035776.htm (accessed 13 February 2009).

Disability Discrimination Act (DDA) (2005) Available online at www.legislation.gov.uk/ukpga/2005/13/contents (accessed 20 March 2011).

Dohrenwend, A (2002) Serving up the feedback sandwich. *Family Practice Management*, 9(10): 43–9.

Duley, J (1980) *Learning Outcomes: The measurement and evaluation of experiential learning.* Washington, DC: National Society for Internships and Experiential Education.

Dunn, R and Dunn, K (1999) *The Complete Guide to the Learning Styles Inservice System.* Boston, MA: Allyn and Bacon.

Eaton, L (1995) A clinical evaluation tool that gives students feedback. *Nurse Educator*, 20(3): 9–10.

Elcock, K (2006) Wake up and learn. *Nursing Standard*, 20(49): 61.

Elcock, K (2007) Where there's smoke. *Nursing Standard*, 21(44): 61.

Elcock, K, Curtis, P and Sharples, K (2007) Supernumerary status: an unrealised ideal. *Nurse Education in Practice*, 7: 4–10.

Eraut, M (2006) Editorial. *Learning in Health and Social Care*, 5(3): 111–18.

Fitzpatrick, J, While, A and Roberts, J (1996) Key influences on the professional socialisation and practice of students undertaking different pre-registration nurse education programmes in the United Kingdom. *International Journal of Nursing Studies*, 33(5): 506–18.

Flanagan, J, Baldwin, S and Clarke, D (2000) Work-based learning as a means of developing and assessing nursing competence. *Journal of Clinical Nursing*, 9: 360–8.

Fleming, J and Courtney, B (1984) The dimensionality of self-esteem II. Hierarchical facet model for revised measurement scales. *Journal of Personality and Social Psychology*, 46: 404–21.

Ghaye, T and Lillyman, S (eds) (2000) *Effective Clinical Supervision: The role of reflection.* Salisbury: Quay Books.

Ghaye, T and Lillyman, S (2008) *The Reflective Mentor.* London: Quay Books.

Ghaye, T, Cuthbert, S, Danai, K and Dennis, D (1996) *An Introduction to Learning through Critical Reflective Practice: Self-supported learning experiences for healthcare professionals.* Newcastle upon Tyne: Pentaxion Press.

Glover, P (2000) 'Feedback. I listened, reflected and utilized': third year nursing students' perceptions and use of feedback in the clinical setting. *International Journal of Nursing Practice*, 6: 247–52.

Gray, M and Smith, L (1999) The professional socialization of diploma of higher education in nursing students (Project 2000): a longitudinal qualitative study. *Journal of Advanced Nursing*, 29(3): 639–47.

Gray, M and Smith, L (2000) The qualities of an effective mentor from the student nurse's perspective: findings from a longitudinal study. *Journal of Advanced Nursing*, 32(6): 1542–9.

Haidar, E (2007) Coaching and mentoring nursing students. *Nursing Management*, 14(8): 32–5.

Harvey, T and Vaughan, J (1990) Student nurses' attitudes towards different teaching/learning methods. *Nurse Education Today*, 10: 181–5.

Hayes, A (2006) *Teaching Adults.* London: Continuum.

Honey, P and Mumford, A (1989) *The Manual of Learning Opportunities.* Maidenhead: Peter Honey Publications.

Honey, P and Mumford, A (1992) *The Manual of Learning Styles.* Maidenhead: Peter Honey Publications. Peter Honey Publications would like us to note that this publication is now out of print but has been replaced by: Honey, P and Mumford, A (2006) *The Learning Styles Questionnaire, 80-item version.* Maidenhead: Peter Honey Publications. Page references in this book relate to the 1992 edition.

Honey, P and Mumford, A (1995) *Using Your Learning Style.* Maidenhead: Peter Honey Publications.

Howard, S (1993) Accreditation of prior learning: andragogy in action or a 'cut price' approach to education? *Journal of Advanced Nursing*, 18: 1817–24.

Jarvis, P (1992) Reflective practice and nursing. *Nurse Education Today*, 12(3): 174–81.

Johnson, D and Preston, B (2001) *An Overview of Issues in Nursing Education.* Department of Education, Science and Training, Australia. Available online at www.pandora.nla.gov.au/pan/23224/20020121-0000/www.detya.gov.au/highered/eippubs/eip01_12/fullreport.htm (accessed 20 March 2011).

Kelly, C (2007) Students' perceptions of effective clinical teaching revisited. *Nurse Education Today*, 27: 885–92.

Kelly, D, Sharples, K and Elcock, K (2007) Take direct action. *Nursing Standard*, 21(22): 61.

Kilbourne, B (1990) *Constructive Feedback: Learning the art.* Toronto, Ontario: Ontario Institute for Studies in Education.

Kilminster, S, Cottrell, D, Grant, J and Jolly, B (2007) AMEE guide No 27: Effective educational and clinical supervision. *Medical Teacher*, 29: 2–19.

Knowles, M (1984) *Andragogy in Action.* San Francisco, CA: Jossey-Bass.

Knowles, M (1989) *The Making of an Adult Educator.* San Francisco, CA: Jossey-Bass.

Knowles, M (1990) *The Adult Learner: A neglected species*, 4th edition. Houston, TX: Gulf.

Knowles, M, Holton, E and Swanson, R (1998) *The Adult Learner*, 5th edition. Houston, TX: Gulf.

Knowles, M, Holton, E and Swanson, R (2005) *The Adult Learner*, 6th edition. London: Elsevier.

Kolb, D (1984) *Experiential Learning: Experience as the source of learning and development.* Mahwah, NJ: Prentice Hall.

Li, S, Chen, P and Tsai, S (2008) A comparison of the learning styles among different nursing programmes in Taiwan: implications for nursing education. *Nurse Education Today*, 28: 70–6.

Lofmark, A and Wikblad, K (2001) Facilitating and obstructing factors for development of learning in clinical practice: a student perspective. *Journal of Advanced Nursing*, 34(1): 43–50.

London, M (1995) Giving feedback: Source-centered antecedents and consequences of constructive and destructive feedback. *Human Resource Management Review*, 5(3): 159–88.

MacLeod, M (1995) What does it mean to be well taught? A hermeneutic course evaluation. *Journal of Nursing Education*, 34(5): 197–203.

Maitland, I (1995) *Motivating People.* Guernsey, CI: The Guernsey Press.

Maslow, A (1943) A theory of human motivation. *Psychological Review*, 50: 370–96.

Maslow, A (1987) *Motivation and Personality*, 3rd edition. New York: Harper and Row.

McMillan, M and Dwyer, J (1990) Facilitating a match between teaching and learning styles. *Nurse Education Today*, 10: 186–92.

Mezirow, J (1983) A critical theory of adult learning and education, in Tight, M (ed) *Education for Adults: Educational opportunities for adults*. Beckenham: Croom Helm in association with the Open University.

Mullen, P (2007) Use of self-regulating learning strategies by students in the second and third trimesters of an accelerated second-degree baccalaureate nursing programme. *Journal of Nursing Education*, 46(9): 406–11.

Murphy, K and Atkins, S (1994) Reflection with a practice-led curriculum, in Palmer, A, Burns, S and Bulman, C (eds) *Reflective Practice in Nursing: The growth of the professional practitioner*. Oxford: Blackwell Scientific.

Myers, I (1995) *Gifts Differing*. Palo Alto, CA: Consulting Psychologists Press.

Myers, I, McCaulley, M, Quenk, N and Hammer, A (1998) *MBTI Manual: A guide to the development and use of the Myers-Briggs Type Indicator*, 3rd edition. Palo Alto, CA: Consulting Psychologists Press.

Nursing and Midwifery Admissions Service (NMAS) (2007) *Statistical Report 2007*. Available online at www.nmas.ac.uk (accessed 28 October 2008).

Nursing and Midwifery Council (NMC) (2004) *Standards of Proficiency for Pre-registration Nursing Education*. London: NMC.

Nursing and Midwifery Council (NMC) (2007) *Essential Skills Clusters for Pre-registration Nursing Programmes*. London: NMC.

Nursing and Midwifery Council (NMC) (2008a) *The Code: Standards of conduct, performance and ethics for nurses and midwives*. London: NMC.

Nursing and Midwifery Council (NMC) (2008b) *Standards to Support Learning and Assessment in Practice: NMC standards for mentors, practice teachers and teachers*. London: NMC.

Nursing and Midwifery Council (NMC) (2009) *Guidance on Professional Conduct for Nursing and Midwifery Students*. London: NMC.

Nursing and Midwifery Council (NMC) (2010) *Standards for Pre-registration Nursing Education*. London: NMC.

Pattison, D, Parsons, D and Weatherhead, C (2000) Connecting reflective practice with clinical supervision. In Ghaye, T and Lilliman, S (eds) *Effective Clinical Supervision: The role of reflection*. London: Quay Books.

Pearce, C (2004) Giving and receiving feedback. *Nursing Times*, 100(50): 46–7.

Pugh, B (1992) Feedback in clinical teaching. *Nurse Educator*, 17(1): 5–7.

Rogers, C (1983) *Freedom to Learn for the 80's*. London: Merrill Publishing Company.

Rogers, J (2007) *Adults Learning*. Maidenhead: Open University Press.

Royal College of Nursing (RCN) (2005) *Guidance for Mentors of Student Nurses and Midwives: An RCN toolkit*. London: RCN.

Royal College of Nursing (RCN) (2007) *Guidance for Mentors of Student Nurses and Midwives: An RCN toolkit*. London: RCN.

Russell, T (1994) *Effective Feedback Skills*. London: Kogan.

Salomon, G and Perkins, D (1989) Rocky roads to transfer: rethinking mechanisms of a neglected phenomenon. *Educational Psychologist*, 24: 113–42.

Schön, D (1983) *The Reflective Practitioner*. New York: Basic Books.

Sharples, K (2006) Shifting priorities. *Nursing Standard*, 21(8): 61.

Sharples, K (2007a) Are you just the job? *Nursing Standard*, 21(40): 61.

Sharples, K (2007b) Sign for success. *Nursing Standard*, 21(51): 64.

Sharples, K (2007c) Supporting nursing students. *Nursing Standard*, 21(50): 64.

Sharples, K and Kelly, D (2006) A hard day's night. *Nursing Standard*, 21(4): 61.

Sharples, K and Moseley, L (2010) Learning to learn in practice: an evaluation of a 35-day practice orientation programme. *Nurse Education in Practice*, 10(2): 57–63.

Sharples, K, Kelly, D and Elcock, K (2007) Supporting mentors in practice. *Nursing Standard*, 21(39): 44–7.

Smedley, A (2007) The self-directed learning readiness of first year Bachelor of Nursing students. *Journal of Research in Nursing*, 12(4): 373–85.

Special Educational Needs and Disability Act (2001) Available online at www.legislation.gov.uk/ukpga/2001/10/contents (accessed 20 March 2011).

Spouse, J (2003) *Professional Learning in Nursing*. Oxford: Blackwell Science.

Steves, A (2005) Improving the clinical instruction of student technologists. *Journal of Nuclear Medicine Technology*, 33(4): 205–9.

Stryjewski, G and Slonim, A (2002) Who says you're too tired? *Critical Care Medicine*, 30(10): 2396–7.

Sung, K (2006) Literature review on self-regulated learning. *Singapore Nursing Journal*, 33(2): 38–45.

Timmins, F (2008) *Making Sense of Portfolios: A guide for nursing students*. Maidenhead: Open University Press.

Tuning (2009) *Subject Specific Competences*. Available online at http://tuning.unideusto.org/tuningeu/index.php?option=content&task=view&id=139&Itemid=166 (accessed 20 March 2011).

UK Central Council for Nursing Midwifery and Health Visiting (UKCC) (1986) *Project 2000: A new preparation for practice*. London: UKCC.

UK Central Council for Nursing Midwifery and Health Visiting (UKCC) (1999) *Fitness for Practice: The UKCC Commission for Nursing and Midwifery Education*. London: UKCC.

Vernon, M (1969) *Human Motivation*. Cambridge: Cambridge University Press.

Watson, R, Stimpson, A, Topping, A and Porock, D (2002) Clinical competence assessment in nursing: a systematic review of the literature. *Journal of Advanced Nursing*, 39(5): 421–31.

Wiggins, G (1998) *Educative Assessment: Designing assessment to inform and improve student performance*. San Francisco, CA: Jossey-Bass.

Wilkinson, C, Peters, L, Mitchell, K, Irwin, T, McCorrie, K and Macleod, M (1998) 'Being there': learning through active participation. *Nurse Education Today*, 18: 226–30.

Windsor, A (1987) Nursing students' perceptions of clinical experience. *Journal of Nursing Education*, 26(4): 150–4.

Withnall, A, McGivney, V and Soulsby, J (2004) *Older People Learning: Myths and realities*. Leicester: NIACE.

Yong, V (1996) 'Doing clinical': The lived experience of nursing students. *Contemporary Nurse*, 5: 73–9.

Young, P (2000) 'I might as well give up': self-esteem and mature students' feelings about feedback on assignments. *Journal of Further and Higher Education*, 24(3): 409–18.

Zimmerman, B (1995) Self-regulation involves more than meta-cognition: a social cognitive perspective. *Educational Psychologist*, 30: 217–22.

Index